THE ALPINE SUN QUARTZ LAMP

IRRADIATION WITH

THE ALPINE SUN QUARTZ LAMP

INCLUDING

SOME ACCOUNT OF LUMINOUS HEAT RAYS

BY

Dr. HUGO BACH

Geh. Sanitätsrat, Dresden

WITH THE ASSISTANCE OF

Dr. FERDINAND ROHR

AUTHORISED ENGLISH EDITION.

Edited by R. KING BROWN, B.A., M.D., D.P.H.

Medical Editor, British Journal of Actinotherapy and Physiotherapy.

SLOUGH:

THE SOLLUX PUBLISHING Co.

PRINTED IN GREAT BRITAIN BY KING AND HUTCHINGS, LTD.,
UXBRIDGE AND EALING.

CONTENTS

LIST OF ILLUSTRATIONS

INTRODUCTION

IN previous editions, the aim of this work was to give a short summary of all that was worth knowing concerning the Alpine Sun Quartz Lamp. The extension which light therapy has undergone during the course of years makes it, however, essential to include, in addition to ultra-violet light, some account of the other rays of the spectrum, particularly the luminous heat rays. These have therefore been so far taken into consideration as the material under discussion renders necessary.

Light therapy is based either upon the application of natural sunlight or the use of artificial sources of light. Among the latter, for ultra-violet therapy the Alpine Sun quartz lamp, designed by Bach and Jesionek, and the water-cooled quartz lamp designed by Kromayer, rank as unsurpassed ; whilst for hyperæmia therapy the Sollux Lamps of Oeken and Cemach.

Ultra-violet radiation produces erythema of the skin ; luminous heat rays only a local hyperæmia.

The distinction is therefore made between ultra-violet therapy and hyperæmia therapy.

The field of use for any source of light is defined by its spectrum. Natural and artificial sunlight must, however, be different in their effects from the outset, since with natural sunlight the influence of atmospheric pressure, temperature, conductivity, absolute and relative humidity, and air movement also come into account. Although these factors are lacking with artificial sunlight, yet the action of the latter upon the human body is nevertheless so powerful that it has attained wide use in therapeutics.

With all physiotherapeutic methods, among which light therapy must be classified, the external covering of the skin is the point of attack. The various physiological functions of the skin, its powers of absorption, transpiration, secretion of fatty matters and perspiration, regulation of bodily warmth, functions as a sense-organ, and that property which is designated esophylaxis, make it intelligible that physiotherapeutic measures affect the most diverse disorders of the bodily economy. It cannot therefore be surprising that light therapy has a wide field, and that it is successfully used in all diseases where the organism as a whole may be benefited by this specific stimulation of the activity of the skin. This is particularly so with ultra-violet radiation. The following pages are written in the hope that they may present a clear account of the subject.

Part I.

ULTRA-VIOLET THERAPY.

Sunlight.

To understand the subject of quartz light, it should be realized that sunlight is composed of rays of different wave-lengths. Each wave-length corresponds to a certain colour or shade. The mixture of colours gives white light.

If a ray of sunlight is passed through a glass prism, it is split up into its component rays, visible to our eyes as the colours of the rainbow (red, yellow, green, blue, violet). The colour band of the sun's rays dispersed through a prism is termed the " spectrum."

The wave-lengths of the rays diminish from red towards violet, so that the red rays are longest, and the violet shortest, in wave-length.

Outside both the red and the violet of the visible spectrum occur rays which are invisible to our eyes ; the infra-red (beyond the red) and ultra-violet rays (beyond the violet). In wave-length, the former are longer than red ; the latter shorter than violet.

The long-waved red and infra-red rays distribute heat, the shorter-waved luminous heat rays penetrate deeply ; the short-waved violet and ultra-violet distribute little or no heat—on which account they are termed cold rays, in contradistinction to the heat rays—are easily absorbed, and do not penetrate deeply.

The wave-lengths of radiations comprising the visible spectrum (red to violet) extend from about 7,000 to 4,000 AU ($1\text{AU} = \frac{1}{10,000,000}$mm.), and those of the invisible ultra-violet rays from 4,000 down to 1,000 $\mu\mu$ and beyond.*

Quartz Light.

Since light-therapy has learned to distinguish the specific effects of the different kinds of light which make up the spectrum, attention has been particularly directed to the long-waved red rays

---

*The Ångstrom Unit is commonly used as a measure of wave-lengths. The various units are as follows :—

1 micron $\quad = 1\mu \quad = \frac{1}{1,000}$ mm.

1 millimicron $\quad = 1\mu\mu = \frac{1}{1,000,000}$mm.

1 Ångstrom Unit $= 1\text{AU} = \frac{1}{10,000,000}$mm.

1

and the short-waved blue rays.   Above all, the rays situated to the right of the violet, in the spectrum reproduced on page 12, *i.e.*, the ultra-violet rays, have outstanding chemical and biological properties which are used with success for medical purposes of the most varied kinds.

When Finsen laid the scientific foundations of light therapy for local diseases, he ascribed the success achieved with his concentrated, cold light to the blue-violet end of the spectrum. Carbon arc light, which he used, has however the disadvantage that its arc contains only a small amount of ultra-violet rays, that it can never be used on more than a small area at a time, and that on account of its weakness in ultra-violet the duration of single treatments must be very prolonged.

Attempts were therefore soon made to devise a source of light more suited to ultra-violet irradiation, and it marked a great advance when Kjeldsen, a Dane, introduced the Dermo Lamp, an iron arc, into therapeutics.   This gives a large output of blue, violet and invisible ultra-violet rays, far exceeding that from the carbon arc.   Treatment with ultra-violet rays could not, however, develop its far-reaching successful results until the mercury vapour lamp was discovered.   Dr. Arons, in 1892, discovered the electric light arc generated in a vacuum tube between mercury poles, giving a peculiar bluish-green light ;   and subsequently, Cooper Hewitt, an American engineer, constructed the first usable mercury vapour lamp.   This developed ultra-violet rays in abundance, but they could not be adequately applied, as the arc was enclosed in a glass envelope which was only slightly transparent to ultra-violet.   Attempts were made by the firm of Schott and Co., of Jena, to obviate this defect by using Uviol glass ;   but only in 1905 was the problem solved by Dr. Küch, physicist to the Hanau Quartz Lamp Co.   After laborious investigation he succeeded in finding a process for fusing quartz crystals into clear pieces, and in constructing a quartz burner from the quartz glass thus produced ; this was the origin of the Hanau-Hanovia Alpine Sun quartz lamp. The radiation from this lamp is intensely rich in invisible ultra-violet, to a degree which is not even approached by any other means known in technology.   Its spectrum, from which the red rays are lacking, shows ultra-violet extending beyond wave-length 2000 A.U., and probably reaching down to 1500 A.U. ; whereas the visible spectrum extends only as far as 4000 A.U.

In 1906 the Hanau Quartz Lamp Co. introduced the first water-cooled quartz lamp. During the next few years, this was used almost exclusively in surgery and in treating skin diseases, *i.e.*, in local conditions according to the method stated by Finsen. During the course of time, particularly after its improvement by Kromayer, it has won an unchallenged place in these branches of therapeutics.

For general treatment, ultra-violet radiation has only been used since 1911. Its injurious effects (*e.g.*, inflammations of the skin, such as occurred at the foundries of Creuzot in Paris and Colonna in Moscow, which Dr. Malakoff traced to these rays) were at first a barrier to their therapeutic use. The fact was, however, established by Dr. Rollier of Leysin, as previously by Dr. Bernhard of St. Moritz, that the mountain sunlight baths with which he achieved such success in treating tuberculosis, particularly of bones and joints, were effective chiefly through their abundance in ultra-violet rays. Only then did practitioners resort to general treatment with these rays from artificial sources. Attempts had previously been made to attribute the action of sun baths to the ultra-violet rays present in sunlight. Since, however, the short-waved ultra-violet rays of sunlight are in great measure absorbed by the denser layers of the atmosphere, and are consequently present only in small amount in the sunlight of lowland regions, the specific ultra-violet action of sun baths was long disputed. Even in 1903 Rieder maintained that sun baths were effective solely through the red heat rays, and the assertion was not directly controverted. With the introduction of the Hanau quartz lamp all doubt was cleared up, as with this artificial illuminant it first became possible fully to study the action of ultra-violet rays, applied as general irradiation, on the human body.

The air-cooled quartz lamp designed by the author, following on his first publication* dealing with general irradiation with quartz light, was brought on the market by the Hanau Quartz Lamp Co. in 1911. It is suited for any sort of treatment with ultra-violet rays.

Down to about 2800 A.U. the ultra-violet rays may be termed mild in their biochemical action ; the shorter ultra-violet rays are sharper in their effects. The most effective rays for therapeutic use extend from 4000 or 3500 A.U. downward. According to

*Deutsche med. Wochenschrift, 1911, No. 9.

Hausser and Vahle* the most effective zone of radiation lies between wave-lengths 3100 and 2800 A.U., although this cannot yet be accepted as certainly established. On the other hand, the fact is cogent that the action of the lamp is very greatly weakened by interposition of the Uviol blue glass filter,† although the filter passes the zone from 3100 to 2800 practically unweakened. Comparison should be made with the spectra given on page 12.

Although sunlight is the most natural and the mildest source of ultra-violet rays, the Alpine Sun quartz lamp is more advantageous in irradiation for therapeutic purposes on the following grounds :—

1. The sun does not shine constantly.

2. The ultra-violet rays of sunshine are for the most part absorbed by the denser layers of the atmosphere, and are therefore only available in adequate amount and intensity in the pure air of mountain regions, when the sky is clear.

3. The Alpine Sun quartz lamp can be used at any time, and anywhere where electricity is available.

In medical journals, both in papers and editorial comments, the opinion is constantly encountered that the ideal artificial source of light would be one which imitated as exactly as possible natural mountain sunlight in all its properties, its spectrum, and its action. Practitioners readily fell back on the use of the carbon arc lamp, because its spectrum shows the same image on a photographic plate as that of the sun. In this attempt to improve on quartz lamps in respect of the action of their radiation, two errors are repeatedly made.

In the first place, the fact is overlooked that a lamp which had in fact entirely the same properties as natural sunlight would be worthless in practice, as thereby only the same results could be attained as Bernhard and Rollier have so splendidly achieved at St. Moritz and Leysin. In other words, the cure of patients would necessitate a full year, or more, of irradiation administered every day and for several hours. Such long times of treatment with artificial light are, however, plainly impossible in practice.

Furthermore, it is again overlooked that the showings of the photographic negative are only qualitatively correct, but not

---

* *Strahlentherapie*, vol. xiii., No. 1, pp. 41-71.
† See pages 10 and 12.

quantitatively, as the shades of black on which conclusions are based are reproduced with uncertainty. Solar radiation ends about the critical region of 3000 A.U., when measured on a silver-bromide negative, or at about the same point as a carbon arc lamp or overrun filament lamp. It cannot be deduced from the photograph of the spectra that mountain sunlight is still very strong in ultra-violet rays about 3000 or 2950 A.U., whilst the carbon arc is almost dark in this decisive region of the spectrum. Yet a lamp which is much poorer than sunlight in the critical zone cannot of course ever be as effective as the sun itself ; and it has already been shown that sunlight in our latitudes is in any case too weak for practical use in healing.

For both reasons, successful therapeutic results can only be expected from the carbon arc lamp if its quantitative output of ultra-violet rays is increased by every possible means so as to approximate to the ultra-violet radiation of the quartz lamp. Owing to the properties of the carbon arc, this is only possible by using currents of enormous strength. Such carbon arc lamps, almost equalling quartz lamps in their therapeutic results, are used in the Finsen Institutes ; in particular, the powerful lamps, of recent fame, used in Scandinavian countries, which consume 40 to 70 amperes of current, connected in parallel on 110 volts direct current. Such powerful carbon arc lamps, like quartz lamps, give splendid results ; and in the domain of surgical tuber-culosis may outclass a single quartz lamp in their effects, since in addition to their output of ultra-violet, which is adequate owing to the enormous current consumption,* heat rays are also simul-taneously produced in great amount. This is doubtless an advan-tage of these powerful arc lamps over the Alpine Sun quartz lamp, with its small current consumption of only $2\frac{1}{2}$ to 4 amps., whose light contains very little luminous heat radiation, almost the entire current being expended in producing ultra-violet.

The question, whether the powerful carbon arc lamps are on

---

* The current consumption of the above carbon arc lamps is :—

$$40 \times 110 = 4400 \text{ watts.}$$
$$\text{or } 70 \times 110 = 7700 \text{ watts.}$$

Against which, the current consumption of the quartz lamp is :—

$$4 \times 110 = 440 \text{ watts.}$$

Reckoned in KW. hours (B.T. units) ⎱ carbon arc = $8\frac{3}{4}$d.
      at 2d. per unit ⎰ quartz lamp = $\frac{3}{4}$d.

To which the large expenditure on carbon electrodes, which are being constantly used up, must be added.

this account preferable to the quartz lamp, must be answered in the negative, as there are many defects and inconveniences in using carbon arc lamps, which are not encountered in the quartz lamp.

The entire manipulation of the carbon lamp, the constant need of handling dirty carbon electrodes, is unpleasant and troublesome. The carbons burn away and need periodical replacement, an unpleasant task entailing waste and frequent breakage, which all goes to increase the estimated costs per burning hour in no small degree. Again, the carbons, which are usually impregnated with metallic salts, burn in the air of the room ; this is also the case with enclosed arcs, although the action is not so rapid. The products of combustion—carbonic acid, carbon monoxide, vapourized salts and nitrogen compounds*—pollute the air. With small ineffective lamps one has to make the best of this, but with large outfits of the kind described above an escape chimney is necessary for the combustion gases, which means that the lamp must be kept in one fixed spot, and is no longer mobile.

The arc is seldom as uniform and constant as the mercury vapour arc ; it often hisses and flickers, discharging glowing particles for which a splutter tray must be provided. This, and the entire arrangement of the carbon arc lamp, preclude irradiation vertically downwards, which is the best method of treatment in most cases. The greater part of the light from a carbon arc is given out horizontally.

So-called " non-burning " open arc lamps have lately been introduced, in which the light is again produced by carbons fitted with cores of salts or metal, e.g., zinc ; this gives the light more of a whitish-blue tone. The spectrum of this lamp ends as high as 3000 A.U. Even in the region just above 3000 it is very weak on the photographic plate. When it is remembered that effective ultra-violet radiation only commences below 3100 A.U., which is the absorption limit of common window glass, the only possible conclusion is that the effective ultra-violet radiation of this lamp must be extremely scanty. To advertise the " non-burning " action of these lamps as none the less an ultra-violet action is liable to cause confusion of ideas, which are already sufficiently chaotic. Light action which is " non-burning," and

---

*Carbon arcs, as is well known, are used in specially constructed furnaces for the direct manufacture of saltpetre.

which therefore does not involve erythema-production, has nothing whatever to do with ultra-violet therapy, but is wholly and solely a light-action. Light sources of such nature, however, do not come into comparison with an actual source of ultra-violet radiation, such as the Alpine Sun quartz lamp, but come under the category of luminous heat-ray sources. Luminous heat rays produce " a splendid hyperæmia, of very deep penetration and long duration "* ; and the therapeutic results from such hyperæmia lamps are excellent in local irradiations. The hyperæmic action of the open arcs described is, however, greatly surpassed by that of the Sollux lamp, which is, further, far superior in convenience of application and ease of handling, as it needs no renewals of carbons or any other attention.

Enclosed arcs (the arcs used for " sun-printing ") are carbon arc lamps with a glass envelope, of which many are marketed under various designations—the "Aureol " lamp, " Heliol " lamp, and so on. With these, only a very weak action can be achieved, on account of the strong absorption by the enclosing glass. From considerations of cost, the envelope cannot be manufactured of quartz, or even of Uviol glass, as this would make the outfit too dear. Recourse is, therefore, had to other kinds of glass, more or less approaching Uviol glass in their nature, but which pass the line at 2800 A.U. only faintly, whereas Uviol glass transmits this almost unweakened. The very necessary narrow band between 2900 and 3100 A.U. is weakened in the same proportion, since a filter never cuts off sharply. Furthermore, the entire radiation is greatly weakened through the unavoidable deposits which form on the glass cover ; and the cleaning of the latter, which often gets broken, is another burdensome matter. For all these various reasons, the use of the enclosed arc had to be given up in favour of open arcs.

In order to achieve effects approximating to those from the quartz lamp, the energy input had to be increased more and more, and to-day powerful arcs are in use operating at the intensities stated above, which correspond to an energy of 5-h.p. When current may be obtained cheaply, as from hydro-electric sources, this may be disregarded ; otherwise, the enormous consumption of current, added to the high costs of carbons, is a factor to be carefully considered in running costs.

*Dr. Oeken (Leipzig).

The inevitable but unnecessary high output of heat rays, against a comparatively poor production of ultra-violet, characteristic of the carbon arc, can hardly be considered a desideratum. A good light-erythema, which can be produced without the slightest difficulty when using the quartz lamp, can only be achieved with difficulty with the carbon arc. With the latter, one is always close to the line which divides a burn-erythema (*i.e.*, a simple burn of mild degree) from the entirely characteristic latent light-erythema produced by the quartz lamp, of which no trace can be seen at the time of treatment and which only sets in some hours later.

Although the value of the light-erythema is still denied by a few, and ignored by many, yet practice shows daily and irrefutably that, apart from the good results of a local hyperæmia, general curative effects, definite and indisputable, from irradiation of the whole body, are only produced by such lamps as also produce good erythema. In fact, the power to cause an erythema, when used for general irradiation, is the sole reliable index of the curative value of a therapeutic lamp, if it is anything more than a hyperæmia lamp, local in its action. This conception has been postulated and emphasized particularly by Prof. Dr. G. A. Rost, of the Freiburg University Skin Clinic, in numerous publications.*

The Alpine Sun quartz lamp is, however, still the sole source of radiation which completely satisfies this proviso. No arguments to the contrary can withstand informed criticism.

Its chief advantage is its incomparably powerful ultra-violet action, especially when burners are renewed in due time, also that this effect can be regulated, by variation of distance, dosage, and use of filters, to suit all cases encountered in practice.

It is another question whether ultra-violet radiation alone is sufficient in all cases.† Here the fact seems to emerge more and more clearly that in many instances the action of ultra-violet rays, good in itself, can still be improved if combined irradiation with luminous heat rays from the Sollux lamp and ultra-violet rays from the quartz lamp is administered, so that the action is a combination of erythema and hyperæmia. This is in accordance

---

Deutsch. med. Wochenschrift, 1915, No. 39. *Ibid.*, 1918, No. 27. *Ibid.*, 1919, No. 46. *Dermatologische Wochenschrift*, 1920, No. 9. *Strahlentherapi⸲*, vol. x., 1920, No. 2. *Ibid.*, vol. xiii., 1922, No. 3. *Ibid.*, vol. xvi. 1923, No. 1.
†Bier and Kisch.

with the theory stated in 1916 by Hagemann and Heusner, the originators of the Sollux lamp.

The application of long-waved heat rays in conjunction with the short-waved ultra-violet, in a measure which is correct and not too great, can be well and effectively carried out by this combined irradiation, *i.e.*, by simultaneous use of the Sollux Lamp, which gives out luminous heat rays in great amount and in an ideal manner. The apparatus is most economical in current ; the consumption amounts to only 1 B.T. unit for the large (Oeken) and 0·33 for the small (Cemach) lamp. As the current consumption of the largest quartz lamp (the Jesionek lamp) is still less (0·77 B.T. units), simultaneous use of the quartz lamp and the Sollux lamp, with its regulated heat action, is far more advantageous than the production of low intensity ultra-violet and of unregulated, excessive heat-radiation from one and the same source of light, as with the carbon arc.

Only those unaccustomed to the use of the quartz lamp can object thereto on the grounds that its action is too strong, especially when the burner is new. The expert, on the other hand, will know how to suit the action to each case by means of lamp-distance, filtration, and time-dosage, and thus avoid undesirable by-effects. It will always remain a great advantage of the artificial Alpine Sun, that results are reached in a fraction of the time required with natural sunlight.

Furthermore, burns caused by quartz light in consequence of incorrect dosage are innocuous ; permanent harm never follows. The burns may best be compared with the so-called " glacier burn " of high altitudes. It follows that the patient is never exposed to injury from quartz light irradiation, such as often arises from incorrect dosage of X-rays. Ultra-violet and X-rays cannot be compared in respect of their effects, as their frequencies are of entirely different ranges. Injuries from X-rays are indeed successfully treated by means of ultra-violet radiation.

Light Filters.

By filtration of light is understood the separation of specified regions of the spectrum through certain interposed media. Filtration of light was introduced by Kromayer. He first used, as the most simple means, cooling water coloured with methylene blue in his quartz lamp, to separate out the irritant rays and produce

B

a deeply penetrating light, especially for treating lupus. The method was, however, unsatisfactory on grounds of cleanliness. He then experimented with a methylene blue filter in front of the lamp, based on the Finsen water lens, and later set an Uviol blue glass instead of the quartz window in front of the lamp, which put an end to the troubles connected with the use of aniline dyes. The dark window, however, became unbearably hot when used for long treatments, and for this reason Kromayer transposed

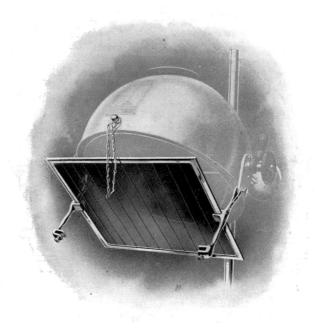

Fig. 1.

The Uviol Blue Glass Filter, for the Alpine Sun Quartz Lamp
(shown attached).

it into the middle of the lamp, so as to lie in the cooling water between the burner and the quartz window; this arrangement has worked well. By this means blue light which is entirely cold can be applied continuously for hours; *e.g.*, in the treatment of lupus.

When, at a later date, the Alpine Sun quartz lamp designed by the author came into use, similar filters were used with this outfit. Uviol glass, however, is a peculiar glass, very difficult to melt, which cannot be manufactured in large pieces. After much spectrographic research, the Quarzlampen Gesellschaft adopted the device of an Uviol film, consisting largely of gelatine, which was entirely similar to Uviol glass in respect of transparency to radiation ; in regard to durability, however, it was not very satisfactory. For this reason the former unsuccessful experiments with Uviol glass were resumed after the war, and it finally became possible to manufacture this in larger pieces ; it is now used in the Uviol blue glass filter.

This special glass completely absorbs the bright yellow and green lines of the quartz lamp spectrum (*see* spectrogram, page 12). The transmitted light thus looks very dark violet to the eye, and its effect on patients is mild and soothing. It passes the effective ultra-violet rays almost unweakened down to wave-length 2800 A.U.

The former Uviol film could never be more than an incomplete substitute for this glass. The latter is now made in strips each about 250 × 25 mm., which are assembled in a metal frame, as shown in the illustration.

The new Uviol blue glass filter can be attached to the lamp hood in two different positions, as shown in Fig. 1 ; one for the open hood, the other when the hood is closed. As it can be turned about the points of attachment, it is easily adjustable to any direction of radiation from the hood ; *e.g.*, horizontally forward or vertically downward.

The filter frame can be readily unscrewed at one side, to allow of renewal of single strips of the blue Uviol glass, in the event of breakage.

In many cases of general and local irradiation with quartz light the blue filter can be dispensed with, and it is usually preferable to utilize the stimulative action of the shortest-waved rays and thus accustom the skin gradually to prolonged irradiation : König, for example, has extended treatment for special purposes up to four hours ; a period which does not come into consideration for ordinary use. For many branches of treatment, however, it is of special importance to cut out the short-waved rays. Jesionek* thus recommends use of the blue filter for the irradiation of wounds when granulating well, since intensive light rich in short-waved

*Münch. med. Wochenschrift, 1915, No. 9.

ultra-violet rays has the property of killing cells. Destruction of cells and tissue is, however, only aimed at until healthy granulation sets in.

FILTERS AND THEIR SPECTRA.

In order to present more clearly the action of filters various spectra are reproduced here (Fig. 2), which are explained below :—

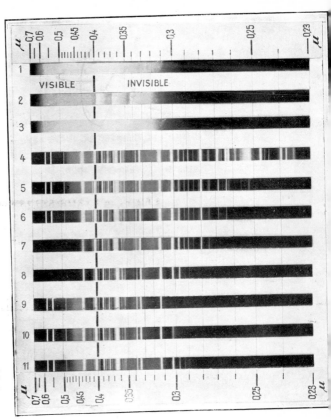

FIG. 2.
Spectra of Different Sources of Light.

The solar spectrum (band No. 1) extends, in our latitudes, down to wave-length 3200-3100 A.U.

The carbon-arc spectrum (2) and Sollux lamp spectrum (3) extend just about as far. A closer boundary cannot be defined, owing to the gradual diminution of intensity toward the shorter-waved rays.

The spectrum of the quartz lamp, unfiltered (4) shows very powerful radiation in the short-waved ultra-violet down to 2300 A.U. The spectrum extends considerably below this point, but could not be reproduced on the spectrograph used.

Through interposition of clear Uviol glass of 1·3 mm. thickness (5) the short-waved end of the spectrum is extinguished to about 2600 A.U.

Double thickness of Uviol glass (6) raises the absorption to about 2700 A.U. (between 2600-2800).

Band No. 7 shows the changes in the quartz lamp spectrum produced by the normal blue Uviol glass filter. At the long-waved end the two bright lines between 5000 and 6000 (green and yellow) are completely extinguished. The light has thus entirely lost the ineffective yellow and green, whose brightness is only disturbing ; and in the visible region above 4000 it only retains the blue and violet portion (which comprises chemico-biologically active rays), and thus appears dark blue to violet in colour. The most valuable ultra-violet region between 2800 and 3200 is unweakened. At line 2800, which is still very strong, the radiation ends ; and this is just what is required by practitioners who work with filters.

Band No. 8 is taken with the same filter in double thickness. The last line is about 2970, which produces a very mild radiation, even more closely resembling that of natural sunlight, but has the disadvantage of the latter, that it entails very long exposures.

Band No. 9 shows the absorption through very thin window glass (only 1 mm. thick). It is seen that only long-waved and comparatively inactive ultra-violet radiation is transmitted. With a normal glass of 2-3 mm. thickness line 3130 is also lost, which means that the radiation has lost all biological action. It is common knowledge that any kind of light rays transmitted by window glass is ineffective. From the absorption spectrum of glass the conclusion may be drawn *a posteriori* that the special healing action of ultra-violet can only begin about wave-lengths 3200-3100.

Bands 10 and 11 show the absorption of thin sheets of celluloid and mica, 0·25 and 0·05 mm. thick respectively. These filters, formerly made for experimental purposes, are neither reliable nor durable in practice. They again show that the correct transparency of the Uviol blue glass filter is scarcely attainable by other means.

Just as, with visible light, it is a familiar fact that the long waves of red and yellow are weak in photography, whilst blue and violet are strong, so also ultra-violet rays of different wave-lengths differ in their effect on the human skin. Rays between 4000 and 3000 A.U. have a mild and slow action, but the far end of the spectrum, which reaches down to 1500 A.U. (although the spectrograph cannot reproduce this), is sharp and irritant. Between 3000 and 2000 there is a gradual transition from the mild to the sharp action. By means of the Uviol blue glass filter the short-waved end of the spectrum can be cut off with absolute certainty about 2900 to 2700 A.U., as shown by the spectrogram.

Jüngling designates the rays above 3000 A.U. penetrative rays, and those below this point, irritant rays.

According to Friedrich Bernhard* the wave-lengths around 3000 A.U. are those which the skin most strongly absorbs. Those around 6000 A.U. are the wave-lengths for which the skin is most transparent to light. This is also the region of the spectrum to which the retina is most sensitive.

IRRADIATION AND ITS TECHNIQUE.

The action of quartz light on the skin, and on the organism generally, is purely biological or bio-chemical. It is produced by irradiation, *i.e.*, by local irradiation of the focus of disease when this is a local condition, or general irradiations for general conditions. As well as the external skin, the nostrils, auditory meatus, mouth and vagina are often treated by irradiation.

Of the three medical quartz lamp models, that made to Kromayer's design is used only for local irradiations. With this lamp the use of quartz rods for treating cavities of the body is also possible. The other two quartz lamps, *i.e.*, the Alpine Sun of Bach, and the Jesionek Quartz Lamp, serve both for general and local irradiation. Further details of these lamps will be found in Part II. Concerning their installation and so forth, full particulars are given in the instructions sent out by the manufacturers

*Münch. med. Wochenschrift, April 4th, 1924.

with all outfits. Here it is only needful to state the practical procedure as below :—

When newly started the burner burns with a bluish and not over-intense light. During the first few minutes the mercury boils fairly strongly from the right-hand negative (cathode) pole, which is the most reliable evidence that this is correctly connected.

Five to ten minutes after the burner is tilted the lamp reaches its full brilliancy, which now remains constant. No after-supervision of any sort is necessary. With the Alpine Sun, in order to curtail the time of burning-in as much as possible, it is advisable to close the hood completely during the first five minutes ; this is, of course, impossible with the simplified models. Irradiation should not be commenced until the burner has reached its full brilliance, or the effect cannot be accurately checked.

During this period the patient is brought into the most suitable posture under the lamp, the position being checked by opening the hood for a brief instant.

It must be remembered that rounded surfaces of the body, such as the shoulders, are readily subject to unequal and over-powerful light action, since the effect of radiation in places where it strikes perpendicularly is often many times more powerful than where its incidence is angular. In general irradiations, the mistake is often made that certain parts of the patient's body, e.g., the knees, are much closer to the lamp than the abdomen. The result is that over-exposures occur on the near points, whilst no reaction takes place on the more remote areas.

Articles of clothing which exclude ordinary light are opaque to ultra-violet also. When treating women, care should be taken lest the rays penetrate unnoticed through blouses of thin texture or open mesh.

The eyes must be protected against ultra-violet rays by means of goggles or dark cloth which is opaque to light. As ultra-violet rays striking the eyes cause painful inflammation of the conjunctiva, it is strongly recommended, as an invariable rule, that every person within five yards of the lamp when in use should be provided with goggles. Not only direct radiation, but the reflection from bright surfaces, e.g., white underclothing on a patient, may cause conjunctivitis or unpleasant irritation with long exposure (from 5 to 30 minutes). Goggles of clear glass are also adequate to protect the eyes, and are less inconvenient, particularly when it is necessary to make observations or take notes during a treatment. Minor parts of the body, such as the ears, are best shielded by covering with protective ointment.

Heusner's Curtain Stand is a particularly excellent means of shutting out distant radiation. It consists of a stand with two cross arms, carrying curtains, rotatable and adjustable for height.

Irradiation is best carried out with the patient lying on an easy couch under the lamp. The eyes are protected by goggles, the face and parts of the body which are not to be irradiated covered by draperies. When the lamp is used from the side, the patient sits or stands before it. With prolonged exposures the recumbent position is preferable, in order not to tire the patient.

The lamp should not be restarted for each patient, as I have often seen done, but left burning continuously as far as possible, (1) in order to have the lamp always available at even strength ; (2) because the burner, on account of the high starting current, is more damaged by repeated starting than by continuous burning. During the periods between treatments the hood should be left half open. Precautions should be taken that unauthorized persons do not look into the hood at such times and thus contract conjunctivitis.

The efficiency of the burner in ultra-violet output diminishes with age, quicker than its output of visible light as gauged by the eye. As soon as the burner arc-tube becomes yellowish or brown, the burner must be reconditioned. The difference between a worn-out burner and a new one is so great that all means of gauging exposure are lost ; on this account, burns arise far too easily when a new burner is again used. As far as possible, the burner should not be used over 800 burning hours.

It is not necessary to protect the burner against sudden changes of temperature, e.g., when windows are opened, since fused quartz is insensitive to temperature changes. When the lamp is switched off, it requires no further attention.

The treatment room must be well ventilated.

The area of the body requiring treatment must be directly exposed to the quartz light, without any covering. With the exception of quartz, almost all materials cut off ultra-violet radiation.

The Action of Irradiation on Exposed Areas.

At the commencement of an ultra-violet irradiation nothing is felt. After a few minutes a feeling of warmth is experienced, which gradually increases to a slight pricking in the skin, and may grow to a burning sensation when irradiation is very powerful. If only mild stimulation of the skin is desired, treatment is stopped as soon as a slight feeling of warmth is experienced. More vigorous irradiations are extended until a slight pricking is perceptible. For further details, consult the sections on " Individual Skin-Sensitivity " and " Dosage."

Three to four hours after a powerful treatment the skin becomes reddened (erythema) and a mild sensation of pricking, smarting, or burning persists. Two or three days later these symptoms disappear, the skin-reddening abates and changes into tan. After powerful irradiation the skin peels in large flakes, and very strong treatment may lead to formation of blisters, as with common burns. As the stimulant rays of ultra-violet light penetrate barely $\frac{1}{2}$ mm. deep into the skin, blisters occur only in the outermost layers of the epidermis, and heal without leaving scars.

Smarting and burning from intense reddening of the skin, or from blisters, are alleviated by the application of diachylon powder or soothing ointment.* In the majority of instances, such symptoms disappear early without any treatment. Healing of a skin burn from ultra-violet radiation, and particularly blister-formation, runs its course like any other burn of the first or second degree, but the effect of the former on the organism as a whole is very different from that of other burns, and is to be regarded as a specific effect from ultra-violet rays.

These symptoms are most strongly evident during and after the first treatment, especially when a powerful irradiation is given. With the following treatments, all sensitivity, reddening or blistering, gradually disappear ; yet it should be remembered that when the skin has peeled, the new surface must be irradiated cautiously with weak doses, so as to avoid a fresh burn. Tanning (pigmentation) of the skin increases after repeated irradiations, and with subjects who pigment easily may reach a dark brown hue ; just as with sunburn, this fades gradually, weeks or months later. Only when long intervals occur between treatments, or after very

* The Hanovia Companies supply a curative ointment, " Hanoviol," which is highly commended.

powerful irradiations, where the lamp distance is small and the time extended, is the effect of the first treatment repeated.

Local or general injury from irradiation, even when this is prolonged to the point of blister-formation, need not be feared. Irradiation may be regarded as entirely free from danger, and can be entrusted to trained assistants. It should also be stated that even with an overdose, quartz light can never cause permanent injury to the eyes. The conjunctival inflammations which may occur, as mentioned above, heal in a few days without treatment ; they are, however, painful and should be avoided.

Regarding the histology of light-evoked inflammation, it follows from Keller's researches that the most striking action of ultra-violet consists in a degeneration of the cells in the *stratum mucosum*. This degeneration never affects the cells of the *stratum corneum* or *stratum granulosum* ; yet even the cells of the *stratum basale* do not degenerate to the same extent—at least, not at the beginning—although it may be the case, as over the papillæ, that these lie nearer to the source of radiation than the spinosum cells in the rete, which there undergo degeneration. The basal cells may, therefore, be regarded as light resistant.

Before this degeneration in the *stratum mucosum* is evident microscopically, toxic products of the cells undergoing destruction must already be present, and these actuate the surge of erythrocytes into the capillaries, and still more the leucocytosis in the irradiated area. Observing the degeneration directly, the leucocytes are already in strong surge towards the degenerating cells. Blister formation and pitting on pressure show that much exudation has already occurred.

Keller has also inquired into changes in the skin after the subsidence of an ultra-violet reaction, particularly with regard to the extent of the increase in resistance. He established the fact that after irradiation, even when no visible inflammation has taken place, there is increased resistance to the action of cantharides plaster.

The action of X-rays on skin which has previously been irradiated with ultra-violet is entirely the same as on the normal skin, as regards erythema, reaction, and final pigmentation. These observations, which were consistent throughout, contradict the writings of American authors, according to which very large doses of X-rays can safely be tolerated after ultra-violet irradiation.

Heat rays, administered with the Sollux lamp, showed in each case of four test subjects a distinct difference in reaction between irradiated and non-irradiated skin. Both in degree and duration, the heat-erythema, transitory as it is, was definitely more powerful on the side previously irradiated.

The epidermal cells manifest increased resistance to mustard plaster irritation when previously subjected to ultra-violet irradiation, but the cells of the cutis, and especially the blood vessels, show none.

Some increase of resistance to carbon di-oxide snow from preliminary ultra-violet irradiation was shown in certain cases.

The effect on tuberculin reaction differs according to the manner in which the tuberculin is applied. Subcutaneous reactions show no difference, the resultant papule is of the same size. On the other hand, with inoculation by Von Pirquet's method, reaction on the non-irradiated side was always of greater extent, but appeared to be weaker in intensity, particularly as regards the degree of vascular disturbance from the reaction. When ektebin is rubbed in, there is considerable reduction both in number and size of the blisters formed on the irradiated side, which corresponds to the increase in resistivity of the epidermal cells mainly attacked by this superficial application of tuberculin. Ponndorf's reaction in some cases establishes differences between the irradiated and non-irradiated sides. In short, it may be said of the various tuberculin reactions that they are the more impeded, the more their manner of application damages the epithelium. In this instance, the irradiated epithelium has acquired protection. Diffusion appears to be less impeded, as is shown by the possibility of late reactions.

Reactions due to trichophytin, under similar conditions, are similarly affected.

Morphine, the test substance for the lymphogogic function of the skin, and adrenalin, the test substance for vascular function, do not manifest any uniform change when subcutaneously injected where the skin has been accustomed to light.

Of interest were the tests of two cases of idiosyncrasy, one to iodoform, the other to turpentine. There were no changes in the reactive symptoms when the substance was applied externally after preliminary irradiation of the skin.*

*Strahlentherapie, vol. xvii., 1924.

THE EFFECT OF GENERAL IRRADIATION ON THE ORGANISM.

During irradiation a sensation of tranquillity and equilibrium is experienced, which may increase to the point of drowsiness.

The pulse becomes fuller and more even, and the breathing deeper ; the number of heart beats and pulse, and also of respirations, are unchanged.

After irradiation, the patient has a feeling of freshness and well-being ; his sleep is deeper and more tranquil, and his appetite improved. The pulse is fuller, the heart's action stronger, and breathing is deepened ; the number of heart beats and of respirations per minute is unchanged. Blood pressure is diminished,* and diuresis increased. The red blood corpuscles are unaffected, but the white are reduced.† Both oxidation and reduction in the organism are increased. Wagner, of Graz, explains this apparent contradiction‡ from fundamental laws governing the phylogenetic relations between light and the living organism. Temporary diminution in weight, usually small in extent, observed after irradiation, is ascribed by Grau to changes in the amount of water in the system. The facts of increase of weight in thin subjects, and of decrease of weight in cases of corpulence, after courses of irradiation, are also confirmed on other hands.

According to Rothmann,§ the decrease in blood pressure which gradually sets in after natural or artificial light baths and persists for several days must be considered a sign of depression of tone in the sympathetic system, as the blood-sugar content is lowered with the blood pressure, whilst the sugar tolerance is increased. The hyperæmia in the skin is the result, not the cause, of the sympathetic hypotonicity. The gases generated by the burners of artificial sources of light cause a depression in sympathetic tone which passes off in a few hours.

The comparative lymphocytosis and the eosinophilia after light has acted on the skin may also be regarded as a symptom of the diminished tonicity of the sympathetic system.

Strongly pigmented subjects do not react. The disappearance of tyrosin from the blood circulation during the course of light treatment is construed as indicating that the tyrosin is retained in the skin as the formative agent in pigmentation.

*Bach, Lampé.
†Berner.
‡*Allgemeine Med. Zentralzeitung*, 1914, No. 17/19.
§Inaugural Dissertation, Giessen, 1923.

The readiest assumption to account for the increase in tyrosin-content of the blood after strong light-inflammation of the skin, is that the inflammation is accompanied by proteolysis and consequent expulsion of tyrosin from the skin.

The hypotonicity of the sympathetic system is a direct result of this, the action of light being developed, indirectly or directly, on the nerve terminals of the sympathetic in the skin. Through the generalized sympathetic hypotonicity the way is opened to the formation of adrenalin, and thus the commencement of pigmentation is made possible.

The depression of function of the sympathetic system leads to powerful hyperæmia of the organs, and can thus be significant from the therapeutic standpoint. Since light therapy, as already stated, may be conceived as a stimulation therapy, it should be noted that the increased gravitation of the red blood corpuscles to the internal organs present in tuberculous cases may be increased still further by light action.

According to Lazarus, relaxation of the vascular system occurs as the result of irradiation in angioneurotic conditions, arteriospastic symptoms, and paræsthesiæ arising from vaso-motor disturbances. This beneficial result also goes to show that there is direct action on the sympathetic system.

The following is extracted from Strahlmann's Thesis (Giessen, 1916) :—

" Concerning the action of light on the nervous system and muscles, it was established by Moleschott as far back as 1855 from experiments on frogs that those animals which were kept in the light had greater powers of response to nerve-stimuli, and greater muscular capacity, than those kept in the dark. With human beings, also, a visible and striking effect can be observed from irradiation both with sunlight and with the Alpine Sun quartz lamp. Even after a few irradiations the patient experiences a feeling of freshness and well-being, the pulse becomes fuller and more even, the respiration slower and deeper. He feels more cheerful, and stronger also, for hours after the light bath. With observation over long periods, it is easily seen how the tissues gain in turgor, and the entire muscular tone, which in phthisical subjects exhibits the characteristic slackness—Stiller states this as a typical symptom of the ' *habitus asthenicus* '—is built up.

" Concerning the action of the Alpine Sun quartz lamp on

bacteria, it may be assumed, taking tuberculous peritonitis as an example, that we have here a case of direct bactericidal deep action of the ultra-violet rays.

" The researches of Buchner and Finsen show that light has bactericidal power ; that ultra-violet rays have this property in special measure was shown by Strebel and Dieudonné. The latter found that light when deprived of ultra-violet radiation lost about a third of its bactericidal power.

" With deep action, however, these bactericidal powers of light are ineffective. According to Klingmüller's investigations, this power is exhausted even in the superficial layers of the skin. The assumption of deep bactericidal action is therefore untenable.

" The action of the Alpine Sun quartz lamp must therefore be of other nature, rather indirect. The inflammatory reaction of the tissues evoked by insolation, producing strong vascular enlargement and increased exodus of leucocytes, must play a large part. In Jesionek's phrase, the leucocytes appear to be influenced in some ' positive, chemotactic ' manner and thereby enabled to render the bacteria innocuous. The symptoms of this inflammatory tissue reaction are powerful hyperæmia and serous exudation, and Jesionek states that these are by no means confined to the surface immediately exposed to irradiation, but extend deep into the irradiated tissues. ' It is the serotactic power of light of which we make therapeutic use ' (Jesionek). There may thus develop, in the entire area of the irradiated tissue, a considerable increase of oxidation, and consequently powerful stimulation of phagocytic action. The effect of light here is therefore primarily that of an oxygen transmitter. In this manner then the action of light in tuberculous peritonitis may also be conceived ; it may here be merely a case of indirect effect by hæmatogenous means. At best, one could hold with Bernhard that there is indirect injury to the bacterial protoplasm through thermal desiccation.

" How this deep-seated action can be explained in detail may possibly be cleared up by further scientific research.

" In any case, the fact remains that irradiation therapy is effective on the inner organs ; a fact first established by Rollier in the treatment of tuberculosis of the kidneys."

Sobotka* concludes from his own observations that the study

*Studies on the effects of experimentally altering local conditions on the reaction to light of the human skin. *Archiv für Dermatologie und Syphilis*, 1915, No. 1.

of ultra-violet reactions and their subsidence in individual cases may be of assistance in recognizing morbid changes in the skin, and in investigating them more closely (pressure before irradiation, injury from anæsthesia, vitiligo). He states that the production of ultra-violet hyperæmia must therefore be classified among those methods which serve to test the skin in respect of its capacity and manner of reaction. He finds that the special advantage of ultra-violet irradiation over other agencies used in testing the skin consists in the fact that it is very easy to evoke a perfectly uniform reaction over a flat area of the skin.

In the author's view, the action of the artificial Alpine Sun on the organism generally is not a penetrating effect of ultra-violet rays directly on the focus of disease, but an action on the skin functions, which in turn sets up action on the organism as a whole. The existing observations and experience indicate that stimulation occurs affecting particularly the various functions of the skin, and that stimulation of the nerves of the skin, especially of the sympathetic, also appears to play a part.

Observations of blood pressure and blood composition extending over years have firmly established the fact that quartz light treatment has a powerful objective effect on the entire organism, and this will be confirmed by every objective observer who tests the action of irradiation on himself. In spite of this, there are still practitioners who express the view that the Alpine Sun action is merely suggestive. Suggestion naturally plays a certain part with quartz lamp irradiation, as with all therapeutic measures, but its main effects have nothing whatever to do with suggestion, as has been shown beyond a doubt by numerous experiments.

Of fundamental importance in this connection are the investigations of metabolism and blood composition after Alpine Sun quartz lamp irradiation, carried out by Dr. Harry Königsfeld.* He established the following results :—A fair degree of uniformity in the excretions set in during the second and third days after treatment ; on the fourth day there was considerable increase in the metabolism of N, P, S, and NaCl, which was maintained on the following days and even increased for S and P. It was therefore established that considerable increase of the entire bodily metabolism took place under the action of irradiation. The records of bodily weight correspond hereto ; there was an increase of 100-150

*Zeitschrift für klinische Medizin, vol. xci., 1921, Nos. 3-6.

grammes on the second and third days, on the fourth the weight remained unchanged, and on the fifth it diminished by 150 grammes. The course of the appetite was similar ; during the first three days there was ample satisfaction from the food supplied, but constant hunger from the fourth day onward. The increase in metabolism affects primarily the albumen-metabolism ; and the salt-metabolism also indicates increase of albumen-metabolism and decrease of albumen in the body. The increased S. metabolism proceeded entirely parallel with the N. metabolism, also indicating increased albumen metabolism. From the increase in P. metabolism it might be concluded that in the decomposition of albuminous substances in the body, the tissues chiefly concerned were those rich in phosphoric acid. The effect of irradiation was like that of great muscular exertion. All experiments verify this result ; *i.e.*, that the entire bodily metabolism, and above all the albumen metabolism, is increased by irradiation with the " Alpine Sun " quartz lamp.

No effect on the erythrocytes and hæmoglobin could be established ; on the other hand, the leucocyte count increased immediately after irradiation but soon sank again. Only after protracted treatments lasting 50 to 60 minutes did the increase persist until the commencement of the next session. The polynuclear leucocytes and the large mononuclear cells undergo changes from irradiation. These changes in the blood picture are not lasting, and have a tendency to rectify themselves. The leucocytosis is probably of similar nature to the digestive leucocytosis.

Königsfeld found that the blood pressure was usually reduced by the extent of 2 to 8 mm. after irradiation.

The anal temperature was reduced after irradiation by 0·1 to 0·9° C., the pulse slower, fuller, and more powerful ; the latter is probably in part due to the effect of repose during treatment.

Aschenheim and Meyer* found the sole constant change in the blood composition after natural or artificial light treatment to consist in a shift in percentage values in favour of the lymphocyte series.

According to Baumann,† the beneficial action of irradiation cannot be direct, but is only set up by the reaction due to certain injuries to the tissues and cells. He found that in human subjects there is a fugitive and inconstant slight leucocytotic shift in the

Zeitschrift für experimentelle Pathologie, vol. xxii., 1921, No. 1.
†*Ibid.*, vol. xxi., No. 3.

cell-count in favour of the polynuclears, with diminution of the leucocytes.

It must be accepted as definitely established from these researches that the Alpine Sun quartz lamp has an objective action upon metabolism, blood pressure, and blood composition.

F. W. Bovie demonstrated the physiological action of ultra-violet rays from the following experiments* :—He divided 250 chicks of a week old, kept in an empty rearing house, into three groups. The first group was allowed to run in the open during the day, the second were given twenty minutes' irradiation daily with a quartz lamp, and the third received only the sunlight which penetrated the glass roof. At the end of the fifth week the birds in the first and second groups had developed normally, whilst those of the third group had made only half their growth. The short-waved ultra-violet rays of the sun's spectrum were kept back by the glass roof, and the experiment shows strikingly how chicks are dependent on the action of ultra-violet rays for their growth.

Peemöller, in his review,† sums up the action of ultra-violet rays on the organism generally as under :—

There is considerable effect on the regeneration of the blood. Further, a shift in the white blood-cell count occurs during the irradiation, conditioned by the nervous system, and apparently dependent on the intensity of ultra-violet energy applied at the session (leucopenia with small intensities, leucocytosis with greater).

There are also far-reaching effects on the circulation and respiration from ultra-violet radiation, in the sense of decrease of blood-pressure, slower and deeper respiration, and increase of respiratory metabolism, which is particularly pronounced in cases of disease.

The increase in respiratory metabolism, according to Peemöller and Kastner, can also be traced to the action of the erythema-producing rays, and is conditioned by the nervous system.

There is also a great effect on the albumen metabolism. The purin bodies may be further disintegrated to form oxalic acid. It depends on the intensity of the irradiation whether synthesis or disintegration of albumen results.

The action of light is still more pronounced on the carbohydrate

*Boston Medical and Surgical Journal, vol. xxii., 1925, p. 1035.
†Strahlentherapie, vol. xx., 1925.

metabolism, both in health and disease (diabetes). The blood-sugar content is greatly decreased. The urine sugar-content also completely disappears in many diabetic cases.

The metabolism of fats, lime, phosphorus, and salt is likewise more or less strongly affected.

In experiments on animals, increased ferment action in the blood was established after irradiation ; according to Pincussen, this is due to the ferments liberated through destruction of epidermal cells.

Dr. L. C. Donnelly, of Detroit,* concludes from observation of 31,000 treatments with the Alpine Sun quartz lamp that in all probability the vitamins must be regarded as transmuted ultra-violet energy. They comprise an important part of our nutrition, which represents nothing less than collected solar energy. It is therefore logical to draw the conclusion that ultra-violet energy is almost as important as food itself.

He states as follows concerning the action of ultra-violet radiation on animals and men :—

Procreative power and reproduction are assisted.

The maternal milk is increased in quantity and in vitamin content.

Pregnancy is tolerated by the mother without loss of teeth, and without disturbance to the functions of kidneys, thyroid, and internal secretion glands.

Parturition is easier.

The child will be well-developed and better able to resist disease.

The child's growth will be healthy and vigorous, and the changes of puberty will come naturally without trouble.

The resistive forces of the body against infection are increased by ultra-violet, even when the diet is low in vitamins, as it regulates the mineral requirements. Speedier growth and better differentiation of the bones are produced.

Secondary sexual characteristics develop more normally.

Furthermore, famous American trainers and doctors to athletic

---

* " Some qualities and uses of ultra-violet energy in medicine."—*American Journal of Physical Therapy*, Vol. ii., 1925, No. 8.

teams call attention to the use of ultra-violet rays in training, and he good results produced thereby. Dr. Clough, formerly medical adviser to the Universities of California, Washington, and Portland, and Jack Weber, trainer to the New York Athletic Club, state that ultra-violet radiation has a bracing and strengthening action, and increases stamina and metabolism. The most famous American athletes, they state, would not care to give up the quartz lamp in their training.

This increase of athletic capacity through artificial Alpine Sun irradiation has also won notice in Germany. Among others, Dr. Lohmeyer, medical adviser for the physical training courses at the Naval School, Flensburg-Mürwick, writes that for over a year he has given artificial Alpine Sun irradiation to the candidates at these courses, particularly during the winter months in Mürwick, when the days are murky. The benefits, not to say the necessity, of quartz lamp irradiation for those in training are irrefutable, and it should be known that the training is improved by the shift which occurs towards the parasympathetic functions of the body through the artificial Alpine Sun irradiation, which has the effect of toning up the sympathetic system.

Irradiation with the Alpine Sun quartz lamp, as Ziegler* expresses it, does not originate special powers in the organism, but only strengthens natural vital processes. This shows that we have here to do with a principle of increasing capacity in the broadest sense.

INHALATION OF THE OZONE GENERATED BY THE ARTIFICIAL ALPINE SUN QUARTZ LAMP, AND ITS EFFECTS.

The ozone developed by the quartz lamp can be used for inhalation ; the burner produces this gas in considerable amount (a conversion product from the atmospheric oxygen), particularly just after starting. It is therefore advisable to commence inhalation immediately the burner is started. A very serviceable device for convenient respiration of the ozonized air is the Hanovia Inhalation Funnel, which is provided with shields to exclude radiation, and is used attached to the hood of the Alpine Sun lamp Otherwise, this air may be inhaled through mouth and nose at a distance of 12-16 inches from the lamp, the eyes being

*Strahlentherapie, vol. xiv., 1922.

covered. Such inhalations are prescribed for catarrhal conditions of the upper air passages, particularly hay fever, and also for whooping cough.

Many practitioners have expressed themselves against this inhalation, on account of the possibility of nitrous oxides being formed by the reaction of ozone with atmospheric nitrogen, or mercury vapour from operation of the burner at considerable over-voltage.

Rost is among their number, and refers in his paper* to the researches of Marek.† He points to the fact that " to remain in air containing ozone, such as is stated to be produced by the action of ultra-violet light, is far from innocuous to the organism, and that Marek has experimentally produced grave harmful effects on the entire organism, and especially on the lungs, in guinea pigs through inhalation of ozone." Marek designates ozone a poisonous gas and very injurious to the body. This statement is also made in text-books on chemistry ; e.g., Pinner, as far back as 1881, in his " Repertorium der anorganischen Chemie," states that ozone cannot be inhaled, as it attacks the organs too greatly. This refers, however, to inhalation of pure ozone, whilst (as Pinner goes on to state) ozone in a mixed state is probably beneficial to health. Experience has also taught that any injury from breathing air which has been altered by quartz light is avoided, provided that abundant fresh air is introduced. None the less, for the reasons stated, caution is advisable in making use of this air for therapeutic purposes, a practice which is still recommended by many practitioners.

Inhalation, by nose or mouth, when deep breaths are taken, gives a feeling of freshness and dryness in the mucous membranes of the nose and throat. If unduly protracted, they may be followed by congestion in the head and singing in the ears ; these, however, are soon dispersed by a stay in fresh air or taking a small quantity of alcoholic liquor.

In order to avoid any unpleasant results, it is advisable to practice inhalation with short pauses every three minutes. In this way, inhalations up to a quarter of an hour's duration are well tolerated in every case.

*" On the ' combined ' irradiation treatment of tuberculosis from a dermatological point of view." *Deutsche med. Wochenschrift*, 1918, No. 27.

†*Zeitschrift für Hygiene und Infektions Krankheiten*, vol. lxxxi., 1916.

Esophylaxis.

Erich Hoffmann,* writing on the action of the artificial Alpine Sun quartz lamp on the skin and the organism in general, mentions that Bruno Bloch, in his Inaugural Dissertation at Zurich,† assumes an important biological function of the skin, hitherto little considered, by means of which " the vital internal organs are protected from germs of disease, or at least have only to fight against a comparatively small and weakened part of the infection." Bloch regards this capacity as one of the most important links between dermatology and general medicine. In this regard he bases his argument on the results of modern investigations into the alteration in sensitiveness or allergy of the skin in trichophytosis, tuberculosis, and syphilis ; and emphasizes " that the skin, above all other organs, takes an active part in the manifestations of allergic immunity and supersensitivity, as contrasted with serum immunity in tetanus, diphtheria, etc., in which the blood is the carrier of the protective forces."

Bloch's statements coincide with Hoffman's conception, in which these are applied to the action of irradiation as follows :—" That tuberculous foci situated inside the body can be benefited by the Alpine Sun quartz lamp, may to-day be regarded as proven ; and on the skin the action of general light baths can be directly observed, as shown by Reyn, Rost, and Jesionek, by the effect on lupus foci which were covered with black paper and protected from direct irradiation. Since the effective short-waved rays, as far as we know, penetrate only very slightly, being mainly absorbed in the outermost layers of the skin (epidermis and papillary layer), their action is in my opinion most reasonably accounted for by the theory that they excite a kind of 'internal secretion of the epidermal epithelium,' and thus assist the healing of tuberculosis by the formation or the increase of protective substances."

In Hoffmann's view, new light is thrown on other curative measures by this hypothesis ; e.g., the beneficial effect of " sweat cures " in infectious diseases, and of inunction of mercury and soft soap. Of particular importance as supporting the assumption of an internal protective function is the observation that when the

*" On an internal protective function of the skin (esophylaxis), with observations on the occurrence of paralysis." *Deutsche med. Wochenschrift,* 1919, No. 45.

†Problems of metabolism and immunity in dermatology.

skin is extensively affected with tertiary syphilis or lupus vulgaris, the internal organs are often unaffected. In particular, it is well known that the co-existence of general paralysis and tabes dorsalis with tertiary syphilis of the skin is extremely rare. Significant in this connection appears the contrast of the meninges and lymph glands. The latter react with very great sensitiveness to invading spirochætæ pallidæ, both locally and generally. The glands are thus not breeding foci for the spirochætæ, but rather defensive organs, and owing to their richness in lymphocytes and histocytes play a part in breaking down infection which is probably far-reaching, just as does the skin, which indeed also contains similar cells.

" Just as the skin is of great importance for the general practitioner as the ' mirror of internal disease,' and often enables the experienced observer to make his diagnosis at a glance, so also does it appear to possess a specific biological function (esophylaxis) by virtue of which it is able to produce protective and curative substances which assist the internal organs and nervous system in their fight against parasites and their toxins, and protect them against these.

" This hypothesis may therefore win recognition as a fact not only of scientific but of practical import, and possibly also assist in improving our therapeutic results in the prevention of the later stages of syphilis."

In connection with these observations of Hoffman, the last work published by the late Dr. Breiger* is also of great interest for ultra-violet therapy. In this work, Breiger reports cures of syphilis by the use of the quartz lamp alone without any other kind of medical treatment.

INDIVIDUAL SKIN-SENSITIVITY TO ULTRA-VIOLET RAYS.

Since the action of ultra-violet radiation on the skin is as a rule perceptible only some hours after exposure, and not immediately, special attention should be given to the individual sensitivity of the skin to the rays, in order to avoid wrong dosage. This sensitivity is dependent on the individual constitution of the skin, and may show wide differences. Skins which are thin, poor in fat, pale, or which perspire readily, and also red, non-pigmented skins,

*On the light treatment of venereal diseases. *Münchener med. Wochenschrift*, 1920, No. 35.

react more strongly to ultra-violet radiation than skins which are thick, greasy, heavy, non-perspiring, or perspire with difficulty, and pigmented skins.

It is of special importance to note that skin which reacts poorly can be sensitized to light, by such means as the following :—

1.   Simultaneous irradiation with filament lamps (*e.g.*, the Hagemann ring) with their long-waved red heat rays ; high-frequency treatment ; thermo-penetration ; and especially irradiation with the large Oeken Sollux lamp, lately constructed by the Hanovia Companies for this purpose. (*See* Part II.)

2.   Courses of bathing, particularly of mud baths, owing to their hyperæmic action, which improves the blood supply to the outer layers of the skin.

3.   Certain internal drugs ; *e.g.*, eosin.   Pincussen administers 0·25 to 0·5 gm. eosin about an hour before irradiation.

Gassul* discovered that irradiation with the quartz lamp produced changes in the internal organs of white mice which had been sensitized with eosin after irradiation for a total period of less than one-fourth of that required without sensitization.

György and Gottlieb† increased the effect of irradiation therapy in rickets by eosin administered *per os*, and Kate Pilling‡ reports similar results.   They administered 0·1 gm. eosin (Höchst blue crystal, with 0·5 sacch. alba, in 10 c. cm. water or milk) on the day preceding each irradiation, spreading the dose over three meals.

According to Finkenrath,§ arsenic sensitizes to light as it does to X-rays ; in one case reported, there was almost a three-fold increase in sensitivity.   This writer considers that the reactivity to light and to X-rays have some relation to each other, so that a test of sensitivity to light may assist in preventing injury from X radiation.

4.   Possibly irradiation combined with X-ray treatment, according to König.‖   H. E. Schmidt,¶ and more recently Bacmeister, have recommended this for treating tuberculous conditions, when

Deutsche med. Wochenschrift, 1925, No. 7.

†*Klinische Wochenschrift*, 1923, No. 28.

‡*Deutsche med. Wochenschrift*, 1924, No. 47.

§*Dermatologische Zeitschrift*, vol. xlvi., No. 26.

‖Section on Tuberculosis of Bones and Joints.   Part III.

¶" Kompendium der Lichtbehandlung " Thieme.   Leipzig.

there is an isolated focus of disease in an otherwise healthy subject ; the X-rays being best administered before ultra-violet irradiation is commenced, and then repeated only some weeks later, when the skin has become accustomed to ultra-violet and does not redden any longer but is pigmented.   Prof. Rost, of the Freiburg University Clinic, has worked out a particularly detailed scheme of combined X-ray and quartz light treatment for the irradiation of lupus.

5.   The photo-catalytic effect after a course of iron treatment or the use of chalybeate mineral waters is stated to result in sensitization of the blood to ultra-violet radiation.

Neuberg* showed that the organic components of animal and vegetable cells become sensitive to light when they come in contact with mineral substances (" photo-catalysis ").   In consequence a diminution of the molecules through sub-division occurs, so that the rays develop an action similar to that of the catalytic enzymes. The molecular division allows the formation of substances possessing highest chemical avidity, particularly the highly reactive ketoses and aldehydes.   Neuberg began his investigations on compounds of uranium and iron.   From a large series of experiments on iron compounds, he demonstrated that both inorganic iron salts and organic iron compounds render animal and vegetable cells photo-sensitive in a high degree.   The chemical reactions involved were very complex ;   the iron setting up reciprocal oxidations and reductions, intermolecular oxygen compounds, syntheses, hydrolytic and uricolytic cleavage, and similar actions.   All these reactions were observed most strongly with direct sunlight, less so with diffused daylight, and did not occur at all in darkness.

Leidner† demonstrated that these photo-catalytic processes are also produced by the rays of the artificial Alpine Sun quartz lamp working on the waters of the Bad Elster springs.

6.   Refractory cases of lupus manifest intensive reaction to gold injections (" Aurocantan ") if the focus of disease is sensitized by an inflammatory irradiation (prolonged exposure at short distance) twenty-four hours previously, or if the body is made more receptive

---

*Chemical transformation through various kinds of radiation.   *Biochemische Zeitschrift*, vol. xiii., xvii., xxvii., xxix., xxxix.   Also " On the photo-catalytic effects of the Pyrmont chalybeate waters."   *Zeitschrift für Balneologie*, vol. v., 1913, No. 19.

†On the photo-catalytic effects of the Bad Elster curative waters. *Zeitschrift für Balneologie*, vol. vii., 1914, No. 8.

by a course of general irradiation. In the same way, cases which did not respond adequately to the action of light showed greater reaction to irradiation treatment after the introduction of gold injections.*

Sack† observed that a course of irradiation which terminated before the onset of smallpox strongly sensitized the skin, and activated and mobilized the eruptive process to a high degree.

Von Gröer and Von Jasinski‡ have "established primary lowering of skin sensitivity after quartz lamp irradiation, which owing to its very short duration is often difficult or impossible to detect. Thus a pronounced hyperalgesia *appears* to set in immediately after irradiation, especially after very prolonged treatment and on highly sensitive subjects. These individual differences appear to bear some relation to the duration of the latent erythema period, and agree on the one hand with the changes occurring in the vaso-motor skin reactivity during the latent period of inflammation which are demonstrable by pharmaco-dynamic means, and on the other with the known facts concerning sensitivity to pain and its relation to the development of inflammation."

A detailed account appears in the " Zeitschrift für die gesamte experimentelle Medizin."

Meyer and Amster,§ and also Mayer,‖ have written on protection of the skin from ultra-violet action by means of tannin. Tannin solution or tannin ointment (1-10%) applied to the skin before a quartz lamp irradiation prevented the development of an erythema on the areas so treated. Schindler found that the application of silver nitrate (5%) in spirit (70%), painted on with a brush, protected the skin against erythema. (*See* section on Dermatology.)

PIGMENTATION.

The bronzing of irradiated areas of the skin which develops after subsidence of the erythema, like sunburn (" glacier-burn ") is due to the formation of pigment.

The production and significance of pigment has been investigated

---

*Spiess and Feldt, of the Höchst Dye Works.
†*Münchener med. Wochenschrift*, April 21st, 1922.
‡*Klinische Wochenschrift*, vol. i., No. 14.
§*Klinische Wochenschrift*, 1925, No. 19.
‖*Deutsche med. Wochenschrift*, 1926, No. 35.

and discussed by numerous authors, and the most diverse hypotheses have been put forward.*   In the words of Strahlmann :—
" Whilst some writers are sceptical concerning the significance of
pigmentation for the prognosis (Vulpius) ; or even regard this as
disadvantageous, like Lenkei, who considers it an undesirable
obstacle to irradiation treatment ; other writers (Rollier, Bernhard,
Hagemann, Bach) emphasize the favourable prognosis which an
abundant pigmentation constitutes for the issue of tuberculosis ;
an opinion which had previously been put forward by Von Schrötter.
Doubtless it seems entirely natural to regard the fact of good pigmentation as evidence of specially strong individual resistance and
therefrom to deduce the probability of a favourable outcome, but
no exact evidence for the correctness of this view has yet been
forthcoming.

" If a comparison be made between the pigmentation from
natural sunbaths and that from the Alpine Sun quartz lamp, it
is found that the former is more lasting, whilst pigmentation
after quartz light baths soon disappears again.   This is probably
due to the absence of the other spectrum colours in the quartz
lamp radiation."

Strahlmann's view that the grade of pigmentation is very different in blonde and dark individuals is not confirmed by other
observers.   The degree of pigmentation appears to be influenced
both by the thickness of the epidermis (see the section on " Individual Skin-Sensitivity "), and by the strength of the first irradiation.   If exposures are weak at the outset and increased slowly,
without producing reddening of the skin, it will be noticed that
no pigmentation takes place, or only to a slight degree after many
exposures ; whilst when treatment is commenced and maintained
with strong doses pigmentation always results.   The individual
sensitivity of the skin to light is also a factor.

Krüger states that individuals who tan well usually recover
quicker than those who remain comparatively pale.   On the other
hand, Vulpius holds that even without tanning good results are
obtained provided irradiation is of sufficient intensity.

Thedering† holds that strong tanning after irradiation is a sign

---

*See publications by Meirowsky, Linser, Diesing, Weidenreich, Strahlmann,
Rollier, Finsen, Schmidt, Unna, Janisch, Maas, Neumann, Freund, Busk,
Jansen, Jesionek, Schäpfer, Adler, Riedel, Pacini, and others.

†Quartz Light and its Uses in Medicine.

of high reactivity, and therefore to be regarded as at least a favourable symptom in prognosis.

Keller* draws attention to the contradiction between the macroscopic degree of pigmentation and the histological amount of pigment. According to this, the macroscopic increase of pigment is in part an apparent increase, *i.e.*, a transposition of pigment, and in part a genuine increase of pigment.

More recently Rothmann showed it from his investigations to be a fact, and not merely a hypothesis, that the augmentation in pigment of the human skin after light baths is closely bound up with important metabolic processes and changes in tonicity of the vegetative nervous system (Sympathetic hypotonicity ; decrease in blood pressure and blood sugar content, increased sugar tolerance, and also decrease in tyrosin content shortly before pigmentation becomes visible and the serum lime content increases.

Jesionek's researches seem to have brought the investigations into the subject of skin pigment to a definite conclusion. He summarizes his views on light action and pigmentation as follows† :—

1.   The pigment-forming, constructive, and kerato-plastic effects of irradiation are direct light actions, developed in the epidermis.

2.   The hyperæmic and nutritive effect is an indirect light action ; it also is based on absorption processes which take place in the basal layer, and develops in an indirect manner by means of substances which only unfold their action when they have passed out of the epidermis into the tissues, to and probably into the vascular system, and thus into the nutritive fluid.

3.   The constructive and kerato-plastic effects of light do not develop unless the hyperæmic power of light is simultaneously unfolded.

4.   The pigmenting power of light acts independently of its hyperæmic power.

5.   But the curative effect of pigmentation, its influence on the organism as a whole, the part which we should ascribe to pigment in the economy of the human body, does not manifest itself any more than does the direct constructive and kerato-plastic action

Strahlentherapie, vol. xvi., 1924.
†*Strahlentherapie*, vol. xi., 1920.

of light in the epidermis, unless the hyperæmic action of light is simultaneously effective.

Regarding all questions of light pigmentation, what can at present be stated with certainty is, according to Jesionek.* as follows :—

1.   The melanin produced by light is the product of a light-evoked intracellular metabolic process.

2.   The appearance of the melanin granules within the basal cells constitutes only a phase, the first phase of a process of secretion which is both initiated by light and continued by light.

3.   The second phase of this secretion process comprises :
   (a) The absorption of light by the melanin granules produced by light.
   (b) The transformation of these granules, through this absorption, into a fluid and colourless mass.
   (c) The issuing of this mass from the epidermal basal cells into the metabolism which goes on between basal layer and papillary bodies, and thereby into the blood and lymph circulation.

4.   Melanin is the chemical forerunner of a chemical substance not yet identified, in the body, which we must term the basal cell secretion.

5.   It is this secretion, doubly charged with light-energy, which introduces the absorbed solar energy into the interior of the human body.

6.   The *stratum basale sive germinativum*, the vital and active layer of the epidermis, is the organ which regulates the relation of the human body to light. It is a light-organ ; the organ of bio-chemical relationship of man, and is the point of attack for that light which we have in mind when we speak of the effects of light on the living human body. It is, however, not only an organ for the reception of light, but also for the transformation of the radiant energy of light ; an organ of light-assimilation. It is an organ of secretory character, an organ which we must class on the same plane as the internal secretory glands.

*Verhandlung der VI. Sitzung des Lupus-Ausschusses, 16, X, 1919.

7. The chemical activity of light is one, perhaps the most important, of the stimuli which set up and maintain the secretory processes in the organ.

8. Curative action, which we are inclined to connect causally with light or with the pigment produced by light, can in fact only be activated by the light-evoked decomposition product of the pigment which light produces ; *i.e.*, by a secretion of the basal epithelial cells.

According to more recent investigations by Peemöller,* pigmentation and erythema-formation do not proceed *pari passu*. It is highly probable that the long-waved ultra-violet rays of wave-length greater than 3200 A.U., and even the dark heat rays, are able to produce a pigmentation.

All hyperæmic skin stimuli assist the action of the erythema-producing rays. The maximum pigmentation is probably due to a certain combined action by erythema-producing and heat rays together.

According to Peemöller,* pigment does not protect against ultra-violet rays. Nor does it fill the rôle of a light-transformer, of a sensitizer, or of a healing substance in potent though invisible form as in Jesionek's statement, but can only be considered as a protective device against the penetrating light rays, serving to guard against heat-retention (and subsequent over-heating).

As a prognostic index, good pigmentation can only be regarded as significant when the pigment has mainly been caused by erythema-forming rays.

Protection of the skin against radiation is conditioned by special processes, which can be discerned microscopically either in an extension of the *stratum corneum* and *stratum granulosum* or in a swelling of the *stratum spinosum*. Perthes' hypothesis of a narrowly localized and specific skin-immunity against certain special groups of ultra-violet rays is, according to Peemöller, untenable.

As may be seen from this brief résumé, no unanimous conclusions have yet been reached on all points regarding the pigment produced by light, but all writers agree that a certain importance must be attached thereto.

Strahlentherapie, vol. xii., 1925, No. 10, entitled " The biological effects of light on healthy and sick persons, with special regard to rickets."

DOSAGE.

The dosage of irradiation with the Alpine Sun quartz lamp necessitates precise knowledge both of the strength of the lamp and of the light-sensitivity of the skin ; *i.e.*, of the organism. For the measurement of these, Keller's Erythema Dosimeter, combined with the Skin Sensitivity Gauge, has proved of particular value. Its use is described below.

The purpose of the *Erythema Dosimeter* is to measure, in a mixture of visible and invisible, or, from the biological standpoint, active and inactive rays, only those ultra-violet rays which are decisive in producing the characteristic " light-inflammation " of the skin ; which means, those below 3130 A.U. wave-length. The human skin is sensitive to wave-lengths of a particular region, from about 3130 to 2500 A.U. A reagent which is to represent the skin in its reaction to light must also be sensitive to the same region of wave-lengths and to that alone. Silver chloride paper, which blackens under the action of light, is chiefly altered by the action of erythema-producing rays, but also by visible rays of no biological activity, as is seen from its use as a photographic printing paper in daylight, under visible and biologically inactive rays which have penetrated glass.

The filter devices of the Erythema Dosimeter allow determination of the value of the erythema rays alone, as the value of the biologically inactive rays is measured simultaneously with the value of the total radiation on the photographic paper. The glass filter at the end of the row of filters is so selected, as the result of biological investigations, that it just completely absorbs all the erythema-producing rays. The amount of blackening of the paper under this filter is therefore a measure of the amount of biologically inactive rays given out by a radiant. The uncovered portion of the paper is irradiated to a standard degree of blackening and the necessary time of exposure measured, then the difference between the blackening of the paper under the total radiation and that of the paper under the glass filter is a measure of the actinic value of the erythema-producing rays during the period of exposure. The actinic value of these rays has then to be correlated with their erythema-producing effect. This has been done by experimental comparisons, in which the relations were determined, for as many radiants as possible with varying output of erythema-producing rays, between the blackening values of the paper and erythema formation on the skin. The erythema-producing rays, in these experiments, were again divided into a short-waved and a long-waved group by means of an Uviol glass filter of certain transparency ; as the filters are arranged in the Dosimeter, this Uviol glass filter lies between the glass filter and the normal darkening of the paper.

On the basis of the curve which can be drawn from these individual values, the corresponding erythema value can be reckoned for every combination of blackenings of the paper given by short-waved and long-waved erythema-producing rays. From this can be reckoned the correction factor needed to convert the time of exposure for the combined radiation (*i.e.*, the effective-biological *plus* the ineffective-biological) into the erythema exposure, the measure for the erythema-producing rays alone.*

By means of the Erythema Dosimeter it is therefore possible to measure the erythema dose of any radiant, provided that erythema-producing rays are contained in its spectrum at all, or in sufficient amount. The limits of use of the apparatus are given by the limits of the tables. The ascertained dosage values are biological values, expressed in Alpine Sun Units (A.S.U.), and correspond with sufficient accuracy to the values ascertained by the iodine method,† which is rather more exact, but has its difficulties in practical manipulation.

An A.S.U. is a dose which (leaving out of consideration rare instances of idiosyncrasy or of insensitivity) evokes an erythema on the body of a subject not accustomed to light but does not reach the toxic degree. An irradiation may therefore be commenced without misgiving at one A.S.U. ‡ For the further irradiation of any part of the skin already irradiated, the rule is valid that the dose may always be increased by one A.S.U. provided the new irradiation is given within a week from the subsidence of the erythema. For each week of delay before the new irradiation is given, one A.S.U. must be deducted from the increased dose thus found, until the amount of the initial irradiation is reached.§

*Further details on the use of the instrument will be found in *Strahlentherapie*, vol. xvii., 1924.

†Methods for measuring the effectiveness of radiants producing violet and ultra-violet rays. By Bering and Meyer. *Strahlentherapie*, vol. i. ; *Deutsche med. Wochenschrift*, 1922, No. 11 ; *Strahlentherapie*, vol. xvi., 1923.

‡*Strahlentherapie*, vol. xvi., 1923.

§*Strahlentherapie*, vol. xvi., 1923.

The dose stated corresponds to the sensitivity of the trunk. Local sensitivity is stated below.*

100—75%. Abdomen ; chest ; back ; pelvis.

75—50%. Inside of elbow ; external upper arm.

50—25%. Neck ; forehead ; hollow of knee ; calf ; thigh.

Sensitivity below 25%. Lower leg ; shin ; hands.

Therapeutic irradiation can be administered on a time basis with a standardized lamp. A quartz burner when first taken into use shows a rapid decrease in effectiveness during the first few months, but is more constant later ; dosage should therefore be standardized once a week at first, and later on every fortnight, or once a month.

The Sensitivity Gauge serves to determine the sensitivity of a subject to light on a small area of skin, when hypersensitivity is suspected, and thus to avoid an overdose when a general irradiation is subsequently given, without on the other hand incurring the risk of giving a dose which does not produce the necessary erythema.

The five apertures on the back of the instrument can be successively opened or closed by a sector cover, so that at a test session five test irradiations can be given on small areas close to each other. The apparatus is fitted with a cover cloth and placed on the test area of the skin, preferably the abdomen, the lamp placed at correct distance as used later for irradiation, and the five apertures opened successively at suitable intervals, *e.g.*, $\frac{1}{4}$, $\frac{1}{2}$, $\frac{3}{4}$, 1, $1\frac{1}{4}$ A.S.U. for the lamp used. The apertures may, of course, be successively closed if preferred.

After twenty-four hours the erythema effect should be observed and the irradiation dose fixed accordingly. A very weak erythema may, of course, have already disappeared in this time. A toxic erythema, such as would be unsuitable for general administration, is shown by its bluish red colour, swelling, and ill-defined margin.

These methods are very much simpler than the former actinimeters and photometers. The Fürstenau Actinimeter, splendidly simple in manipulation, is still used by many practitioners. It is, however, unreliable, as according to Keller[†] it is not thereby

Strahlentherapie, vol. xvi., 1923.

[†]The utility of the Fürstenau Actinimeter for Alpine sun treatment. *Deutsche med. Wochenschrift*, No. 17, 1921.

possible, at least, not in the way it was ordinarily used, to determine variations in the effectiveness of the mercury vapour lamp, and the instrument was rather a hindrance as it was misguiding in this respect. The other advantages of the instrument are, of course, not affected by this consideration. It is based on the light-sensitivity of selenium, and therefore reacts only to visible light, primarily to the yellow portion of the spectrum, as practical test confirms.

Among the large number of Photometers, that by Bering and Meyer appears most suited to its purpose, but its manipulation is troublesome in practical use. It applies the photo-chemical oxidation of iodine-hydrogen for the measurement of light-intensity,* and its modification by Rost and Keller deserves special mention, as this was the means by which the Alpine Sun Unit (A.S.U.) was first determined. Keller adopts the erythema of the skin as the biological measure of ultra-violet radiation, holding the view that the therapeutic success of a quartz light treatment goes *pari passu* with the erythema produced, and terms the necessary dose of ultra-violet to produce this erythema on an unaccustomed skin the " Alpine Sun Unit " (A.S.U.). An Alpine Sun Unit is therefore the dose of biologically effective radiation given at a certain distance from an Alpine Sun quartz lamp with unfiltered light. In Rost and Keller's modification it is determined as follows :—

" A beaker of 5 cm. diameter and about 100 cc. capacity is filled with 25 cc. each of two solutions, (a) 1% potassium iodide, and (b) 5·3% sulphuric acid, together with 6 to 8 drops of starch solution about 1% strong and 1 cc., 1 /400 n-sodium-thiosulphate ; *i.e.*, with the same solutions as used in the Meyer-Bering method. The potassium iodide solution must always be prepared fresh, and this is best done by dissolving a quarter of a gram of powder, which has been carefully kept from damp, in 25 cc. of tap water shortly before use. If the liquids are added in the order stated above, the mixture should not turn blue when the starch is added ; otherwise, free iodine has already formed in the potassium iodide solution. The other reagents can be stored for some weeks, and may therefore be purchased as required. The composite reaction liquid is not very stable.

" The freshly prepared solution is placed under the quartz lamp at any selected distance, contained in a beaker of the above dimensions, which is stood for convenience on a sheet of white paper. After some time blue streaks appear on the surface, which must be made to disappear by stirring with a glass rod. The solution itself remains colourless, as is easily seen in the intense light of the lamp, until in one instant a blue colour appears, which deepens rapidly in a few seconds ; the onset of this blue colouring gives the time of reaction. Care should be taken that the entire surface of the beaker is exposed to the rays. An estimation every two or three weeks appears sufficient to standardize any one lamp.

" If the A.S.U. is determined for a quartz lamp at a certain distance in this way, then dosage is given by time at the same distance. A course of irradiation is usually begun with one A.S.U. ; in rare instances with $\frac{1}{2}$ A.S.U. as a precaution, and increased by 1 or $\frac{1}{2}$ A.S.U. each time, after the erythema has subsided."

From these theoretical data, the following dosage may be taken as valid for local and general irradiations :—For the first local irradiation, take 3 minutes duration at a lamp distance of 20 inches from the area to be treated. Each succeeding irradiation is prolonged by 3 to 5 minutes at the same lamp distance and by degrees extended to the maximum exposure of 20 minutes. At the outset, the irradiations should be given at intervals of two to four days. If erythema develops some hours after irradiation, the next irradiation must be deferred until this has subsided. As soon as no further erythema develops, irradiation can be given daily.

With less sensitive skins, a start may be made with 5 minutes exposure at 20 inches distance, and this can be gradually prolonged by 5 minutes at each succeeding treatment up to a maximum of 30 minutes at the same distance. The interval between treatments is regulated as with normally sensitive skins.

With general irradiations, as large an area of the body as possible is exposed, either the entire front or back of the body ; or both sides at one treatment, in succession or simultaneously if two lamps are available. The chest and abdomen, or the back, are also sufficient. Treatment is begun with 3 minutes at one metre distance, and increased by 3 minutes at each successive irradiation up to the maximum of 30 minutes. The distance is decreased at each successive irradiation, i.e., from the second onward, by 10 cms. each time down to the minimum of 50 cms., which should then be maintained for all following sessions.

As a rule irradiations may be given at intervals of two to four days, and even every day on insensitive skins, so long as no erythema results. In all cases it is advisable to make a break of three to four weeks after twelve to fifteen sessions. The skin then again becomes more capable of reaction to ultra-violet radiation. Provided such breaks are adhered to, irradiation may be continued for years.

With powerful general irradiations, given with the object of producing an erythema, it is advisable to irradiate only one side of the body. Each side is thereby afforded a longer interval between treatments, so that the erythema can subside by the next irradiation.

The length of each session, the interval between treatments, and number of sessions in the course are, with general as with local irradiations, dependent on the individual sensitivity of the skin to ultra-violet rays. With general irradiations the lower hood of the lamp must be fully opened.

The dosage for specific diseases is more fully stated in Part III.

If possible, only one patient should be treated at a time ; with little children, two or three together at most. The prime consideration is that cases should be treated individually.

The Jesionek lamp, on the other hand, is excellent for the simultaneous treatment of several persons (four to five adults), particularly if two or more such lamps are placed opposite each other and the patients sit between as then irradiation is given on all sides at once.

On the technique of irradiation with the Jesionek lamp, Prof. Jesionek states* :—

" The intensity of radiation from our lamps is such that exposure of a slightly pigmented blonde for one hour at a distance of 4 metres produces a light *dermatitis erythematosa*. With brunettes, in whom the skin of the trunk shows somewhat higher content of pigment, it requires $1\frac{1}{2}$ to 2 hours exposure for an equal degree of inflammatory hyperæmia. The lamp may therefore be placed 5 to 6 metres from the blonde subject in order to produce nothing more than enrichment of pigmentation after one hour's exposure. The biological zone of the lamp may therefore be estimated at about 6 metres. The length of the treatment room depends on the number of lamps which it is desired to introduce along the

Zeitschrift für Tuberkulose, vol. xxv., 1915, No. 1.

walls, having regard to the conditions of treatment distance mentioned elsewhere (*i.e.*, intersection of the cones of radiation). The longer the treatment room is built, and the more its plan approaches a corridor, the greater the number of patients who can be simultaneously treated."

Thedering irradiates the naked body on all four sides at 1 metre distance, daily to three times a week, and in the sidelong posture he irradiates also the interior of the thighs, so as to secure as even as possible a stimulation of the entire skin organ. He uses clear goggles to protect the eyes, as the conclusions of investigators into the biological action of light show that even the rays entering the visual organ stimulate and assist metabolism.

Only in cases where outside considerations prevent irradiations daily or frequently during the week does he consider it permissible slowly to increase the occasional quartz sun bath up to half an hour. He therefore distinguishes between a general light bath and an ultra-violet douche.

Generally speaking, one may approve Thedering's methods, yet it is necessary to have regard to the light-sensitivity and reactivity of the skin as well as the specific action of radiation, and also to what result is aimed at from irradiation in each individual case. The lamp distance and duration of treatment must therefore be suited to individual circumstances, in order to achieve the primary object, an effective skin-reaction. The practitioner should not, therefore, timidly seek to avoid irritation of the skin, *i.e.*, an erythema ; on the contrary, he should aim at producing it, and the duration of treatment may be extended beyond the normal period without misgiving when skins of less than normal sensitivity are concerned, as there is no cause for anxiety even in a severe skin reaction.

Dosage of irradiation must be increased cautiously and by very slow degrees at the outset, until the skin has become tolerant. An erythema is, however, desirable even after the first irradiation. Precise instructions should therefore be given regarding period of irradiation and distance from the lamp. The difficulty, for patients and attendants, of being sure of distance at any moment when freedom of movement was permitted was solved by Dr. Lippmann, Chief of the St. Georg Hospital in Hamburg. He scratched con-centric circles with a nail in the floor covering (linoleum) at distances of 25 cms. and filled them with white oil paint. The lamps were so placed that the burners stood over circle ○ (*see* Fig. 3). The practitioner is thus able to prescribe the exact distance, and the patients can move freely in the 25 cm. zone between two circles which has been prescribed. With later irradiations, such exact dosage is no longer necessary. Length of dosage, which should be adhered to strictly, is facilitated by the Hanovia Interval Timer, which rings an automatic alarm.

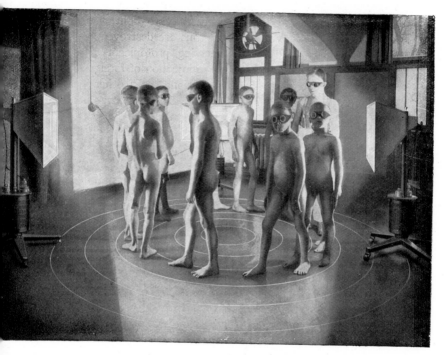

Fig. 3.

The General Ultra-Violet Light Bath (six Jesionek Lamps) at the Poliklinik of the St. Georg Hospital, Hamburg, showing dosage circles marked in the floor. Ten children are walking round the inner circle, whilst the use of the outer circle gives accommodation for fifteen children.

Over-intense irradiation (short lamp-distance, long period of treatment) may result, with individuals sensitive to light, in cerebral congestion, headache, noises in the head, depression and sleeplessness. These troublesome symptoms soon pass off without treatment, or may be overcome by small quantities of alcoholic liquors (brandy, port) and abundant fresh air. Subsequently, a feeling of well-being and freshness, with peaceful sleep, always ensues.

Protein Shock Therapy.

According to the investigations of Nathan and Sack,* it is established that toxic products from degenerated cells are produced in guinea pigs by ultra-violet irradiation. These products evoke vascular reaction ; at least, the primary. The irregularity of this epithelial degeneration permits the deduction that single cells differ in their individual sensitivity to light. In the end, however, entire layers of the epidermis are destroyed.†

This extensive destruction of living protoplasm acts on the organism in the same manner as the injection of foreign albumin ; *i.e.*, as a stimulant like protein injections.‡ In other words, the action of ultra-violet therapy would be the same as that of protein shock therapy.

Ostermann, of Vienna, has conducted very thorough investigations of the local stimulative action of ultra-violet light, of which he has published an account.§ His results are so important for ultra-violet therapy that they are quoted here verbatim :—

" The living cell accepts every unusual exogenous or endogenous stimulus as noxious, and responds thereto by mobilizing its defensive measures, to an excessive extent. Even the smallest stimulus injures the cell, yet it recovers quickly, and in the process uses up only a small part of the mobilized defensive substances to master the attacking forces. Stimulation therapy therefore utilizes the excess of the defensive substances produced, always polyvalent in nature. In addition to the stimulus of the general quartz light bath, which is very different on the individual superficial cells of the skin, there is the general parenteral protein-body effect through absorption of the products of inflammation from the light-erythema, with its general and focal reactions, which are often striking. The field of indications of parenteral protein-body therapy is co-extensive with that for general quartz light therapy, if the latter is intensified by localized erythema doses. Since unduly extensive erythema may let loose undesirable secondary effects (pyrexia, nausea, vomiting, headache, insomnia, cardiac irregularities, and

---

Archiv für Dermatologie und Syphilis, 138 ; 1922.
†Keller. *Strahlentherapie*, vol. xvi., 1924.
‡Van Pée. *Liege Medical*, No. 15, April 13, 1924.
§*Zeitschrift für Erkrankungen des Bewegungsapparates*, 1924, No. 2.

in consumptive patients focal reactions whose extent cannot be foreseen), these local erythema doses should be carefully regulated, with strict regard to the general condition. In any case, before any fresh irradiation, any focal or general reactions set up by its predecessor must first subside ; the temperature should be carefully watched, especially in tubercular subjects."

In general, Ostermann applies, during a course of 20 general quartz light baths, 4 to 6 local doses at 20-10 cms. distance, of 3-5-10 minutes' duration, in addition to the general bath. The local application is made on varying parts of the body (chest, back, stomach, thigh), over an area of one to two palms breadth, so that an intensive erythema with slight inflammatory œdema is produced on this spot, which may develop to *dermatitis bullosa ;* and that during the entire course of light treatment some circumscribed area of the skin is affected by the stimulus of light. The more torpid and chronic the course of the disease, the more energetic and frequent must these light stimuli be (chronic arthropathic and myopathic conditions, neuralgia, surgical tuberculosis, are instances). A suitable treatment is to maintain the skin over localized chronic inflammatory conditions (*e.g.*, tuberculosis, arthritic conditions, etc.), or over those parts of the body of which the local metabolism needs increasing (gouty deposits, alopecia, varicose ulcers, etc.), constantly under the effect of light stimulus, in an area not too circumscribed, so that subsidence of the preceding erythema is not necessary. This gives the transition from general and etiological to local and symptomatic stimulation therapy, with its well-known analgesic and derivative effects. Whilst acute lumbago, pleurodynia, and the like are often relieved by a single erythema dose of 5 minutes' duration at 20 cm. distance (possibly intensified by a Sollux irradiation of 20-40 minutes), the dose has had to be increased up to 60 minutes at 10 cms., given at weekly intervals, in cases of trigeminal neuralgia, sciatica, alopecia, and varicose ulcer (ulcus cruris).

In order to produce the same stimulus on a skin area where the erythema has already subsided, it is necessary to give a dose averaging half as much again as the preceding. The inflammatory pain from the erythema can easily be subdued by soothing ointment,* or by compresses of aluminium acetate on the greased skin.

---

e.g. Rp. Liquor alumini aceti   1%
            Lanolini ana   40
            Vaselini   20

The local erythema doses are doubtless capable of assisting the production of antibodies in the skin, and the importance of these was suggested even by the old-time doctors who only commenced the treatment of syphilis when the secondary exanthema had broken out, and who hailed a heavy exanthema in scarlet fever or measles as a sign that the internal organs had escaped. In pædiatrics, the incidence of tuberculides is counted as of good prognosis for the course of tuberculosis. Metasyphilides are much more frequent in those cases where the skin has evinced only slight syphilitic symptoms. In the modern abortive therapy of syphilis, the aim is to make good the deficiency of natural immunizing processes by parenteral injection of protein bodies ; reactive quartz light therapy is at least equally valuable. Breiger has pointed out the striking good effects of general quartz light irradiation, particularly on tertiary skin syphilis.* Ostermann treated by irradiation, among other cases, one patient with ulcerated gummata of the sternum and clavicle, who could not tolerate specific therapy on account of his very reduced condition. After 20 general and 5-6 intensive local irradiations the ulcers healed completely with soft scars, and the weight increased by 6 kg. Wasserman reaction + + (at the beginning of treatment it was only slightly positive). Specific treatment was now well tolerated, and cure resulted.

The scanty penetration of distant irradiation caused Ostermann to resort to compression treatment with the Kromayer lamp and blue filter in treating obstinate neuralgic conditions, arthritic stiffening of the joints, chronic bursitis, gouty deposits, and the like. Up to publication, his results comprised eighteen such cases, in which he consistently obtained such striking results in a very short time that he recommends this as most suitable for confirmatory tests. A pressure irradiation of only 6-8 minutes' duration produces a deep-penetrating hyperæmia, which persists for days. A few hours after treatment an intensive erythema occurs on an area corresponding to the size of the quartz lens used, and after one to two days the uppermost layer of the epidermis forms a bleb filled with clear serum. One or two such doses are given daily ; with neuralgic conditions, on Valleix's points, and if necessary following the course of the affected nerve, as in sciatica ; with arthritis, on the entire periphery of the joint ;

*Münchener med. Wochenschrift, No. 3, 1920.

with gouty deposits, *e.g.*, on the calcaneum, around the insertion of the Achilles tendon, close to one another. The practitioner's aim should be to press the lens as deeply as possible into the soft parts against the nerves, or into the hollows of the surface of the joint right against the articulation of the joint itself, the patient's posture being regulated accordingly. The lamp must always be held vertical, and the area to be treated must therefore be adjusted to the burner. If a joint, for instance, has had 4-5 such intensive erythema doses within two or three successive days, the result is a vigorous inflammatory reaction and loosening of the joint, during which passive and active mobilizing movements are begun, and which can if necessary be improved by diathermy, mud packs (after the skin has been greased), or parenteral protein. This technique produces the deepest and most strongly active hyperæmia which can be obtained by any therapeutic measures.

As has been shown by Liebesny, both experimentally and clinically, the basal metabolism is greatly increased under the action of general quartz light irradiation. He was chiefly interested in the urea metabolism. With chronic polyarthritic and neuralgic conditions, he was repeatedly able to demonstrate high uric acid content in the blood with normal or even sub-normal content in the urine, and delayed reduction of it even on a purin-free diet ; so that, in his opinion, gout is much less frequently diagnosed in Germany than it actually exists. Under the action of general quartz light baths, intensified by local erythema doses, he was in many cases able greatly to reduce the uric acid content of the blood serum and to obtain abundant excretion of urates in the urine.

None the less—and this applies generally—these very powerful skin stimuli must not be continued *ad infinitum*, as there is a limit to the reactive capacity of the organism. For this reason, the maximum duration of general irradiations should not exceed 30 minutes, and after every twentieth irradiation a de-pigmenting break of several weeks should intervene (" intermittent helio-therapy ").

Procedure could, however, also be according to the following scheme :—Irradiate with the Alpine Sun quartz lamp, commencing with 2-3 minutes on each side of the body at a distance of $1\frac{1}{2}$ metres. Treat every second day at the commencement, keeping the same distance but increasing the time by one or two minutes according to the previous reaction, until the total dose amounts to 30 minutes after about 6 to 8 irradiations. If reaction is very powerful, omit the increase in dosage or allow a day's pause.

During the following treatments the distance is decreased by 10-15 cms. each time down to one metre. At the same time the sides of the body (sidelong posture with outstretched arm) and the pulmonary apices (the patient being seated) are included in the total duration of 30 minutes. From now on the interval is extended by a day each time until the final dose of 30 minutes at one metre, with a seven days' pause, is reached ; this may be continued for months together, and always evokes a mild stimulant action without exhausting the reactive capacity of the organism. With this programme, also, a local erythema dose should be administered from time to time. Physical well-being and increase of weight are the best evidence that the degree of stimulus and reactive capacity are always proportioned to each other. This technique appears suited for chronic articular and muscular rheumatism, rickets, the exudative diathesis, spasmophilia, osteomalacia, atherosclerosis, syphilis, and metabolic disorders (gout, diabetes, corpulence) ; whilst for all forms of tuberculosis where reactive capacity is still present, intermittent heliotherapy is advised.

Ostermann's surmise, expressed as far back as 1913, that ultra-violet exercises a tonic action on the sympathetic system, has meanwhile found powerful corroboration in the demonstrated increase of calcium ions in the blood after general irradiations, since the sympathetic tonicity and blood calcium content run *pari passu* (adrenalin in rickets and osteomalacia). This explains why quartz light courses with calcium and adrenalin, on the one hand, or belladonna or atropin on the other, are often beneficial in pneumogastric neuroses ; such as bronchitis, bronchial asthma, hyperacidity, salivation, mucous colitis, urticaria, nervous dys-menorrhœa, etc. It is conjectured that the cellular injury by the stimulus of light leads to the reactive production of internal secretions (suprarenals, thyroids, ovaries) which increase calcium metabolism. Hence the absolutely specific action of quartz light in rickets, osteomalacia, and the callus formation.

In addition to the technique outlined, of general quartz light therapy intensified by local erythema doses, the action of quartz light can also be assisted by suitable combination methods, and the results still further improved thereby. These include preliminary or simultaneous hyperæmia by means of Sollux irradiation, diathermy, mud packs, etc. ; as well as combination with Thyroidin, iodine, ovarian extracts, Testogan (in chronic polyarthritic conditions accompanying hypothyroidism, at the change of life, or with gouty diathesis) ; internal or venous calcium therapy (Afenil) in rickets, spasmophilia, bronchial asthma, etc. ; parenteral therapy by protein bodies, and suitable dietetic measures (low-purin diet for gouty diathesis, or bronchial asthma ; additional vitamins in rickets ; and the like). The action of photo-dynamic sensitizers is of great interest ; these include chlorophyll, hæmoglobin, hæmato-porphyrin, skin pigment, bile pigment and other fluorescent dyes such as eosin, methylene blue, the heavy metals, etc. If mice, for instance, are injected with hæmatoporphyrin and exposed to sunlight, severe œdema and death quickly supervene, whilst if kept in the dark they are not affected. Hæmatoporphyrin is a derivative of hæmoglobin, traces of which are found in urine even when normal but particularly during fever, poisoning by sulphonal, and hydroa æstivalis. A. Perutz was able to set up hydroa æstivalis in guinea pigs by injecting them with fluorescent dyes which had been irradiated with ultra-violet. Experience shows that minute quantities of the heavy metals (Fe, Hg, Bi, Cu, Ag, Au) in the blood circulation are sufficient greatly to increase the effect of ultra-violet action on the organism (catalytic action), and conversely, the effect of these metals on the organism is definitely increased under the action of ultra-violet radiation. Ostermann repeatedly observed that when accompanied by simultaneous general irradiation there was marked increase in the effect of iron in anæmia, of copper (Lekutyl preparations) in surgical tuberculosis, of gold (Aurocanthan and Krysalgan) in laryngeal tuberculosis ; whilst iron alone, for instance, has no action, and ultra-violet of itself does not affect the red blood cell count. The local light stimuli were obviously increased when combined with subsequent treatment with " copper ointment " (for lupus), with Reimer's heavy metal ointments (for varicose ulcer), and with painting of the mucous membranes with nitrate of silver (precipitation of metallic silver during the irradiation). At the Heidelberg Children's Clinic, under Györgi and Gottlieb, it was found that internal administration of eosin (0·1 blue crystal + 0·2 sugar per day, taken at meals) doubled the action of quartz light treatment in rickets, the duration of cure being reduced to half. He repeatedly succeeded in obtaining striking results in septic processes and influenzal pneumonia by combined treatment with argochrome (methylene blue and silver) given intravenously, or collargol enemas, and general irradiation. In this very domain a great future should be open for light therapy.

Liebermeister, of Düren, also reports* on successes with stimulation therapy by ultra-violet irradiation, which he applied with the water-cooled Kromayer Lamp in cases of tubercular lymphomata and peritonitis. He irradiated areas 10 cms. in diameter at a distance of 1-1½ metres every day ; first treatment 10 minutes, increasing to 15, 20, 25, according to the case in hand. The restricted local erythema had a very speedy beneficial action on the acute symptoms in every case. Favourable changes in the blood picture and the general condition were also observed simultaneously, in almost every instance.

Liebermeister recommends this stimulation therapy for tuberculosis of other organs. Since the irradiated surface is always comparatively small, other areas can constantly be chosen to set up fresh skin action, and the strength of the reaction can be graduated at will. In this way beneficial action on the patient by means of erythematous stimulation of the skin, exactly dosed, can be continued over several months.

This gives us, therefore, in addition to local and general irradiation as hitherto practised, stimulation-therapy in the form of " over-dosed local irradiation."

THE ACTION OF ULTRA-VIOLET RAYS ON FOODSTUFFS.

It has been established by American investigators, Harry Steenbock and Anny L. Daniel,† and confirmed by P. György of Heidelberg,‡ that antirachitic properties are imparted to inert oils and fats, olive oil, cotton seed oil and linseed oil, by irradiation with the artificial Alpine Sun quartz lamp. It was shown by experiments on children that olive oil and milk which had been irradiated with quartz light for one-half to one hour at a distance of 20-30 cms. produced considerable deposit of calcium, and cured florid rickets and tetany without any other medicament, like cod liver oil.

*In the *Fortschritten der Therapie.*
†*Journal of the American Medical Association*, No. 15, 1925. p. 1093.
‡*Klinische Wochenschrift*, vol. iv., 1925, No. 23.

It was further established that various kinds of foodstuffs can be activated in this way by means of ultra-violet irradiation. Particularly suitable are fresh fats, such as butter, olive oil, coconut oil, and so forth ; when old and rancid, this capacity diminishes. Milk, and yolk of egg, are also suitable, as they contain substances capable of activation.

György found that a sample of fine salad oil, otherwise completely odourless, smelt strongly of cod liver oil after brief irradiation with quartz light. If the oil was heated to the point of ebullition before irradiation, it did not take up the odour. The sample which smelt of cod liver oil also manifested the same taste. Pure olein showed neither smell nor taste after irradiation. Irradiated human and bovine milk, both raw and boiled, was characterized by an indefinable, stale, almost mouldy taste and smell, resembling train oil. György was unable to give any satisfactory explanation of this striking phenomenon.

Therapeutic tests of nutrition with irradiated milk gave the following results :—In 16 out of 18 cases, the clinical and blood-chemical manifestations of rickets and of tetany were greatly ameliorated or cured. A special explanation was found for the two refractory cases, so that these need not necessarily be registered as failures. According to György, length of treatment appears to be four to six weeks, but in many cases only a fortnight is needed. With Moro, he designates the change in the milk " jecorization," by which term he also implies that possibly ultra-violet rays and cod liver oil in fact possess a common antirachitic principle.

In a further paper* György states that " the antirachitic radiant energy can also be induced in substances in powdered form, such as wheat flour or chemically pure crystalline cholesterin." He was also able to jecorize milk powder, which was irradiated by quartz light in a thin layer (1-2 mm. thick) from a distance of 30 cms. for three-quarters to an hour, and conserved in tins. The prepared fluid mixture made from such " jecorized " milk powder was characterized by a peculiar, slightly rancid taste and smell, like the jecorized milk although in much smaller degree, but was readily taken by the children and well tolerated.

Such irradiated milk powder can accomplish the complete clinical and blood-chemical cure of rickets, both the florid forms and those without complications, and of tetany, in just the same

*Klinische Wochenschrift, No. 17, 1926.

time as jecorized native fresh milk, with visible deposition of lime as seen by radiograms.

We thus have in this irradiated milk powder, which preserves its induced radiant energy undiminished for at least four months, a durable antirachitic medicine, reliable in its action.

Kurt Brandenburg* is also of this opinion, and regards it as immaterial whether active compounds are administered or whether the carriers of this action are administered and subsequently activated by irradiation.

Of practical importance is the fact that a further field in therapeutics is here opened, since not only rickets, but certain forms of tuberculosis, are also benefited by ultra-violet radiation, and possibly also certain forms of anæmia. It is possible that in this manner the action of immediate irradiation, if not replaced, can yet be intensified by simultaneous courses of diet in which irradiated foodstuffs are included.

Investigations of metabolism on healthy children showed that olive oil irradiated with ultra-violet produced considerable deposit of lime. The latter was just as great as in investigations which were carried out with cod liver oil.

Further experiments showed that the activity acquired by inert oils from irradiation is an entirely permanent property. It was demonstrated, for instance, that olive oil which had been irradiated eleven months previously and kept in a sealed bottle in the dark had lost none of its activity. The oil was irradiated by exposure to the rays of a mercury vapour lamp, in a thin layer at about half a metre distance for half-an-hour. According to Brandenburg, there appear to be many carriers of activation among the natural foodstuffs containing lipoid groups of the nature of sterols. The above-named oils and fats take a leading place, provided that they are fresh.

Hess† succeeded in imparting specific activity to cotton seed oil and linseed oil by ultra-violet irradiation. The daily addition of 0.1 c.cm. of irradiated oil to a rickets-producing diet was sufficient to protect rats from developing rickets. There must therefore be an antirachitic factor present *in vitro*, outside the living organism.

Hess and Weinstock have been able to identify the constituent of foodstuffs which is activated through irradiation as a specific

*Med. Klinik, No. 20, 1925.
†Zeitschrift für Kinderheilkunde, No. 4, 1925.

substance, namely, cholesterol.* Spectroscopic investigations showed that activated cholesterol absorbs ultra-violet radiations to a less degree than does ordinary cholesterol, although with very prolonged irradiation the activated cholesterol becomes even less transparent than non-irradiated cholesterol.

The point of chief importance is that, under the action of light, constituent substances in the cholesterol of the skin fat are constantly split off, and these regulate the skeletal development during the years of growth, and probably play other important parts in the adult metabolism.

Beumer ascertained that there is a decrease in the amount of precipitate, when cholesterol is precipitated with digitonin, through ultra-violet irradiation. His theory is that the antirachitic factor found in the unsaponifiable portion is the same substance which develops from cholesterol under irradiation, and which is shown in this experiment as a loss in the digitonin precipitation.

The antirachitic activation of rickets-producing foodstuffs by artificial Alpine Sun irradiation was checked and confirmed by Serebrijeski, H. Vollmer and E. Zadeck.† Hottinger‡ ascertained that human and bovine milk acquire antirachitic properties from irradiation with ultra-violet light, and that rickety children fed on such milk are cured. Anæmic conditions subsisting with rickets were not affected by the irradiated food, so long as excess of milk was given. Although calcification progressed, there was no improvement in the function of the bone marrow.

Halzac and Nassau§ accomplished cures within three weeks of rickets and tetany in babies with milk which had been irradiated for a very short time (45 seconds), healing being checked by clinical, blood-chemistry, and X-ray observations.

Luminous Heat Rays.

At the other extreme to erythema therapy with the ultra-violet radiation of the artificial Alpine Sun quartz lamp, we have hyperæmia therapy with the luminous heat rays of the Sollux lamp. These rays produce only a hyperæmia of the skin and deep penetrating intensive warming throughout the tissues, just

---

*Beumer on the problem of rickets and the action of ultra-violet radiation upon cholesterol. *Münchener med. Wochenschrift*, No. 38, 1925.

†*Zeitschrift für Kinderheilkunde*, vol. xl., No. 6.

‡*Schweizer med. Wochenschrift*, No. 8, 1926.

§*Zeitschrift f. d. gesamte physikalische Therapie*, vol. xxxi., No. 6, 1926.

as with any other application of heat, but more intensive and without discomfort. When they are applied according to the instructions, skin burns cannot possibly result. If these arise in isolated cases, they are treated as any other burn. This method of hyperæmia treatment is preferable to all others on account of the convenient manipulation and intensive action of the Sollux lamp.

The lamp (more closely described in Part II.) is so adjusted that the diseased focus lies in the centre of the field of light. Before the first treatment, and always with very sensitive skins, the skin should be greased with vaseline. When the face is irradiated, the eyes must be protected by goggles.

The size of the field of light should be regulated according to the extent of the diseased area ; and the distance of the skin from the cork ring, according to the sensitivity of the skin.

A lamp distance of 15-20 cms. has been found suitable for the first irradiation, and 8, 10, 15 or up to 20 cms. for those succeeding.

Duration of treatment should be $\frac{1}{4}$, $\frac{1}{2}$, or up to $\frac{3}{4}$ of an hour for the first irradiation ; later ones, $\frac{1}{4}$, $\frac{1}{2}$, $\frac{3}{4}$ or up to 1 hour.

Irradiations can be administered once or twice daily, or every other day, according to the objects in view and to the sensitivity of the skin.

Artificial Sunlight for Health.

With quartz light, or ultra-violet irradiation, there is a fundamental difference between its use for sick persons on one hand, and for the healthy on the other. *All treatment of disease must remain exclusively the province of the medical practitioner.* It is obvious that quartz lamp irradiation is included here, and must only be used for treating disease under medical advice and supervision.

The case is different with the irradiation of healthy subjects as a precautionary and tonic measure. In this case, provided that the prescribed distances and times of treatment are observed, self-irradiation can be recommended without hesitation. It may be counted among the hygienic measures, such as air baths, sun-baths, physical culture, sports, and hydrotherapy in its most varied applications, which are successfully used for the maintenance and promotion of health without special medical supervision.

Notable in this sense are the observations of Bier in his work " A Doctor's Thoughts on Medicine,"* concerning physical dis-

*Münchener med. Wochenschrift, No. 34, 1926.

harmony. He is of opinion that within the limits of the inherited constitution much can be achieved if the adaptability of the organism is influenced aright, as the ancient Greeks knew. Their aim and achievement was the " Kalokagathia," beauty and goodness of body, or physical harmony ; and beyond this, psychic harmony, and in this aim they availed themselves, among other means, of their outstanding educational scheme of Gymnastics. " Gymnastics " means, literally translated, " naked activity." This name does not only imply bodily exercise, as is usually supposed, but it also expresses the idea that nakedness—*i.e.*, what we understand by air and sunbaths, among which ultra-violet irradiations must be given a prominent place, as will be shown—was the necessary preparation for the Kalokagathia

Bier, like many others, has earlier drawn attention to the great importance, from the medical point of view, of gymnastics in the ancient Greek sense for racial health and development, and urges that this gymnastics—*i.e.*, naked activity—should again be used as a means of healing, as was the case in ancient Greece. In Bier's opinion it would be an excellent remedy for the many forms of physical disharmony, such as corpulence, leanness, physical and mental sloth, clumsiness, awkwardness, stiffness. Moreover, a means which, properly used, could never be injurious.

These remarks of Bier's may be linked up with the very readable paper by Leo C. Donnelly, to which reference has already been made in Part I. of this work. In his treatment room he teaches pregnant mothers that ultra-violet treatment leads to birth of normally developed children, that pregnancy is tolerated without loss of teeth or hair, or development of abdominal protuberance, that kidneys, tonsils, and the inner secretory glands function properly, that the mother is protected against high blood pressure, that her muscular system, including heart and abdomen, will be well developed, and that she will thus be in good condition of body and possess sufficient muscular strength to give her child normal birth. The tone of the lower abdominal muscles will be such that parturition will not result in the development of a large abdomen, her blood coagulation time will be approximated to normal so that she is safe from fear of hæmorrhages, and also, her resistance to infection will be so strong that she has little to fear from infection. He also explains to the expectant mothers that by these irradiations during pregnancy they will be enabled to bring healthy children into the world, who begin their life with a store of light energy and are therefore more resistant to disease, are especially protected against rickets, mainly owing to the fact that they will not suffer from deficiency of calcium and phosphorus in the blood ; further, that the young mother will have healthy, nourishing milk in plentiful amount, so that she will be able to nurse her child without difficulty.

He impresses on the parents of growing children that ultra-violet energy, or quartz lamp irradiation, is of great importance for the development of small children, and that with other children later the onset of puberty, of menstruation, etc., enters in a natural manner and without complications.

These teachings of Donnelly may be summarized as meaning that he warmly recommends prophylactic irradiation at all stages of life ; with babies, for the promotion of growth and protection against rickets ; with growing children during the years of puberty ; with women, during menstruation, pregnancy, and the change of life ; with men, for improving their general health, and also during the climacteric years.

In America ultra-violet irradiations are also used for athletes in training, and it has been shown that their athletic performance has thereby improved.

Prof. Leonard Hill also advocates irradiation for the healthy in several papers, (e.g., B.M.J., Sept. 12th, 1925). In his view, ultra-violet irradiation should be given when solar irradiation is impossible. The lamps should not only be in the hospitals, but also in the schools and public baths ; two to three irradiations weekly being administered as a prophylactic measure, under the necessary supervision.

Various authorities have expressed similar views in Germany. Dr. Bruntaler, Medical Officer of Hildesheim, writes* that his experience justifies the recommendation of quartz light baths as a form of municipal welfare work which deserves further test. If his experience is confirmed, he recommends that a course of artificial Alpine Sun should be included in the school curriculum. Dr. Lohmeyer, Medical Officer to the Course of Physical Training at the Naval School at Mürwick (near Flensburg),

---

*cf. his work, Artificial Alpine Sun courses as a form of municipal welfare work amongst school children. *Jugendfürsorge*, No. 11, 1925.

uses the artificial Alpine Sun in training ; he recommends it particularly for dull days during the winter. Wilhelm Dörr, Second President of the Union of German Sporting Instructors, expresses himself to the effect that " the quartz lamp has the advantage in sport that it affords a means of becoming brisk and fit during the decisive preparatory months of winter, and its wonderful results are seen during training in the summer." Recently, Thedering has expressed the wish that the artificial Alpine Sun should be used in the family circle. In his work, " Sunlight as Healer,"* he writes : " How easy it is to install a hanging lamp in the bathroom ; and what a source of health and vigour for the members, young and old, particularly when delicate children are concerned. The manipulation of the artificial Alpine Sun is so easily learned that any layman could work it without difficulty." Thedering's conviction is that natural and artificial sunlight treatment practised regularly throughout the year would obviate the necessity of many a costly course of treatment in hydropathic establishments.

The use of the quartz lamp for healthy subjects is only in the form of general irradiations according to the technique stated in Part I. of this work. As a rule, two to three irradiations weekly are given, which may be continued for months. Cases are known in which irradiation was successfully continued for years without interruption.

*English edition, Sollux Publishing Co., Slough.

Part II.

INSTRUMENTS.

1. THE ALPINE SUN QUARTZ LAMP.

The Alpine Sun quartz lamp, the first quartz lamp for medical use in both local and general irradiation, was introduced by the writer in 1910. The current model (Fig. 4), improved by better devices for vertical travel and by the addition of a counterweight, has proved excellent in practice. A detailed description of the artificial Alpine Sun quartz lamp will be found in the catalogues issued by the manufacturers.* The essential part of the lamp, the source of radiation, is the quartz burner (Fig. 5), contained inside the hood. This has undergone modifications of shape recently. The hood consists of two hemispheres, of which the upper constitutes the hood proper, whilst the lower serves as a cover, and can be adjusted to any position desired by means of axial rotation, which enables a wide variation of the radiation emitted. Since closing the cover prevents access of air and can thus give rise to great overheating of the burner, which will cause frequent extinction of the burner and wears it out prematurely, it is advisable not to close the lower hood more than is necessary. The lamp can be used either mounted on a stand, or suspended. It is started, after the current is switched on, by tilting the burner.

The Alpine Sun quartz lamp is available in various types, *i.e.*, for direct current of 110, 150, and 200–250 volts, for alternating current from 90 to 250 volts, and again in four different models, as under :—

The Stand Lamp (Standard Model), shown in Fig. 4.

The Normal Suspension Lamp.

The Simplified Stand Lamp.

The Simplified Suspension Lamp.

For use on exceptional voltages, special resistances are necessary.

* In Great Britain, the British Hanovia Quartz Lamp Company Ltd., Slough.

The latest model of the Bach Alpine Sun lamp (Original Hanau-Hanovia) is now built in the improved form shown in the illustration.

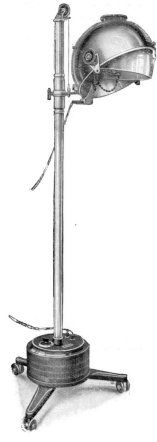

Fig. 4.

The Alpine Sun
Quartz Lamp

Standard Model for Direct Current, with
counterweight in the upright tube.

The weight of the lamp is counterbalanced by a counterweight travelling up and down inside the hollow upright tube.   Counterweight and lamp are connected by a steel cable which is led over a pulley at the top of the upright.

The hood itself, and the burner, remain as before.

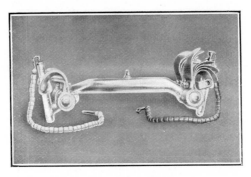

FIG. 5. THE QUARTZ BURNER.
(D.C. type.)

Electrical data for the different burners are as under :—

Circuit Voltage VOLTS	Normal Current AMPS.	Starting Load AMPS.	Voltage across Burner VOLTS	Length of Arc in num. (Approximate)	Photometric intensity of burner CANDLES	Hourly consumption WATTS
Direct Current		Alpine Sun Electrical Data:				
110	4–4·5	11	75	60	1100	500
220	3–3·5	8	150	120	1800	770
	Jesionek Lamp Electrical Data:					
110	6	16	75	60	1800	660
220	3·5–4·5	11	150	120	2700	990
Alternating Current	(Primary)	Alpine and Jesionek :				
110	7·5	11	160-170	120	2250	800
220	3·7	9		(tri-polar)		

With the new arrangement, vertical travel of the lamp is effected with the greatest ease. By means of a milled hand screw at the side of the upright sleeve, the lamp can be clamped at any height.

The resistance on the Direct Current Lamp, and the transformer on the Alternating Current type, are arranged immediately on the feet at the base of the upright.

The castors are very easy running.

2. The Kromayer Lamp.

Whilst the Bach Alpine Sun and the Jesionek quartz lamps serve especially for general irradiation (the Alpine being also used to some extent for local treatment), the Kromayer quartz lamp is exclusively for local irradiation. It was the first quartz lamp for medical use, and has been known since 1906.

Kromayer constructed his lamp with the ∩-shaped quartz

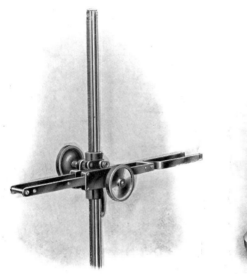

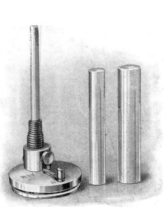

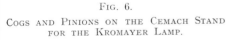

FIG. 6.

COGS AND PINIONS ON THE CEMACH STAND FOR THE KROMAYER LAMP.

FIG. 7.

QUARTZ ROD APPLICATORS, CEMACH PATTERN.

burner contained in a watertight metal casing with a quartz window, inside which cold tap water circulates in order to deprive the radiation of all heat. His lamp has proved excellent in dermatology, as compression treatment with the quartz applicators is thereby made possible.

In gynæcology, dental surgery, and otology also, it has been used for many years, in conjunction with special quartz rods (see Fig. 7) with best results.

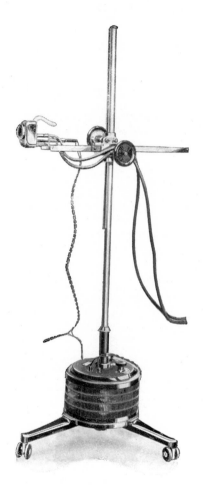

FIG. 8.

THE KROMAYER WATER-COOLED
QUARTZ LAMP FOR LOCAL TREAT-
MENT, ON THE CEMACH STAND.

3. The Jesionek Quartz Lamp.

The Jesionek Quartz Lamp contains a more powerful quartz burner in a large box-shaped reflector (see Fig. 9). Its main use is for general irradiations, which according to modern conceptions are much more important than local treatment for most diseases. Further, with this lamp several patients can conveniently be treated simultaneously. (See p. 43.)

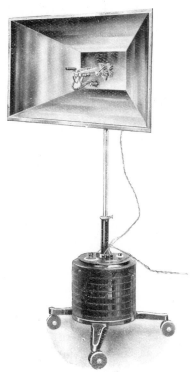

Fig. 9.
The Jesionek Quartz Lamp.

This model is much used in the equipment of large light treatment rooms.

Prof. Jesionek writes concerning the lamp* :—

" The light treatment rooms must be so constructed, and so equipped with lamps and reflecting devices, that they are

*Zeitschrift für Tuberkulose, vol. xxv., 1915, No. 1.

thoroughly filled with chemically active radiation, as evenly distributed as possible, and that the radiation incident on the subjects within four walls, in respect of its biological action, approaches the light out of doors as nearly as is possible by technical means.

"A man in movement undergoes a fairly even irradiation over the entire body only if the light reaches him from the sides and if, in moving, he passes from one cone of rays to another. Physical

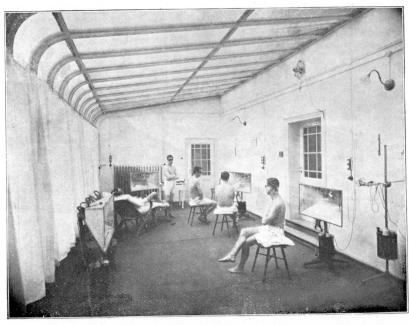

FIG. 10.

IRRADIATION HALL, fitted to Prof. Jesionek's plan, in the Munich Hospital, "Links der Isar."

and biological considerations preclude any other arrangement of the lamps except along the side walls of the room, in such a way that the quartz burners are about the height of the umbilicus of an adult, *i.e.*, about 70 cms. from the floor. If the cones of rays from adjacent lamps cross at a given distance from the wall of the reflector, an approximately even distribution of radiation in the centre of the room will result. The action of this direct ultra-violet radiation from the lamps is intensified by reflected light, an indirect ultra-violet radiation being obtained by finishing the walls, ceiling, and floor of the room with materials which reflect ultra-violet."

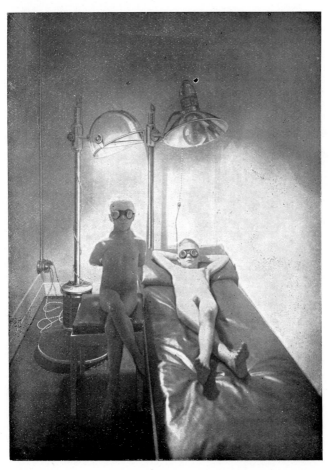

FIG. 11.

Illustrations are given (Figs. 11–13) showing collective and individual irradiation.

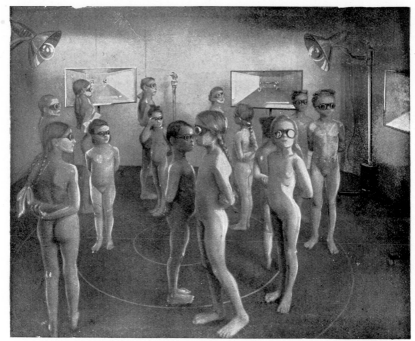

Fig. 12.

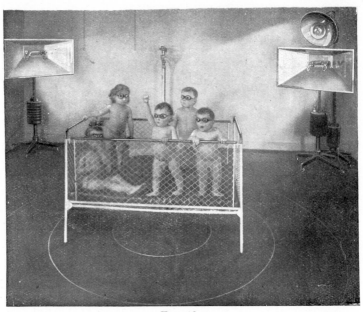

Fig. 13.

4. The Sollux Lamp.

The Sollux Lamp is a very intense heat radiator. It not only renders the skin particularly receptive to ultra-violet radiation, like the Hagemann Ring of filament lamps, but is also of value as an independent therapeutic device in all cases where healing

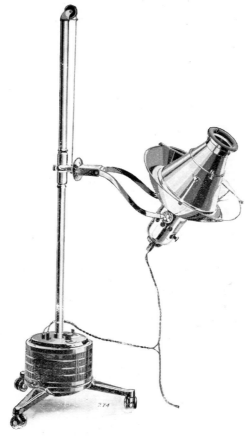

Fig. 14.

The Large Sollux Lamp.—Dr. Oeken Model.

effects can be expected from radiant heat. It gives speedy relief from pain, by prolonged local irradiation using the conical reflectors, in cases of inflammation of the testicles, epididymis, and prostate, in tonsillitis, catarrh of the throat and the nose, inflamed tendon sheaths, stiff joints, discharges from the joints, glands, and sciatica. American writers narrate splendid results in cases of pleurisy and pulmonary inflammation obtained by irradiations of the chest, both front and back, lasting an hour each, using the large parabolic reflector.

Dr. Heusner reports successful results in cases of epididymitis. Spiess and Vogt, of Frankfurt, and Dr. Cemach, of Vienna, in otitis media ; Dr. Gustav Riedel, of Frankfurt, describes excellent results in treating surgical tuberculosis from the combination of the Sollux lamp and the quartz lamp (see Figs. 15 and 16).

Dr. Nürnberg, of Elberfeld, writes* :—

" Results in all cases of septic conditions of the nasal sinuses even after the first treatment, were great relief of the oppression and headache, with strong discharge from the nose. In course of time I have come to rely almost exclusively on the Sollux lamp in treating diseases of the nasal sinuses, with very good results. It would be very good if the use of the Sollux lamp were extensively adopted by specialists, as it constitutes a valuable addition to our scanty therapeutic resources for treating sinus diseases."

The Sollux lamps can be used with red, blue, and daylight screens. With the daylight screen it serves, *inter alia*, for testing medicinal preparations.

The source of light is a special bulb, made under patented special processes on the lines of a filament bulb, filled with nitrogen at two-thirds atmospheric pressure ; the filament is a tungsten wire arranged in a thin spiral with many coils, enabling a heavy current load and thereby intensive radiation. The radiation renders the skin surface soft and hyperæmic, as is necessary for the most effective reception of ultra-violet radiation. The hourly current consumption amounts to one kilowatt only.

The reflector is composed of several parts :—

    (1) The large parabolic reflector itself, containing the 1,000-watt bulb, which has a telescopic focussing adjustment.

Med. Klinik, 1923, p. 240.

In this simple form, the apparatus is used for general irradiation of the body, and as an auxiliary to the Alpine Sun quartz lamp (see Fig. 15).

(2) The rear conical reflector piece, with large aperture, for local irradiation (for the technique of local treatment, see page 55) is attached to the rim of the parabolic reflector by means of the three arms with which it is fitted. The round filter frame, which is provided with

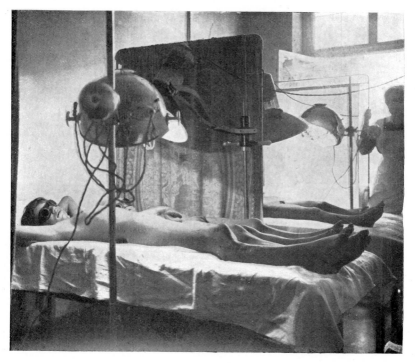

Fig. 15.
Irradiation with the Alpine Sun and Sollux Lamps, in the University Clinic for Orthopædic Surgery, Frankfurt a. M.

lateral openings for ventilation, can be attached before the aperture, and serves to carry the red, blue, and daylight screens.

(3) The front small conical reflector extension serves to concentrate the light on still smaller surfaces. At its opening

a cork ring is fitted, to obviate burns from accidental contact with the hot metal : a space is left between the ring and the reflector itself, for ventilation purposes.

High frequency, diathermy, X-ray and radium treatment can also be successfully combined with quartz light irradiation, but owing to the imperfect state of knowledge of these combination

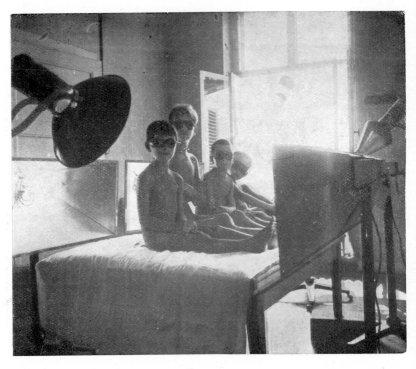

FIG. 16.

Irradiation with the Jesionek Lamp and Sollux Lamps, in the University Clinic for Orthopædic Surgery, Frankfurt a. M.

methods, no attempt will be here made to discuss them more closely. The special works on the subjects should be consulted for further information.

5. THE SMALL CEMACH SOLLUX LAMP.

(Portable Model.)

The small Sollux lamp of Dr. Cemach's design constitutes a very practical outfit. In contrast to the large Sollux lamp designed by

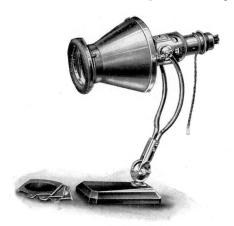

FIG. 17.

Heusner and Oeken, it is only applicable to local irradiation of circumscribed inflammatory processes, particularly for acute conditions of the ear, nose and throat, having been specially designed for this purpose. A ruling factor in its design was the consideration that a special lamp for the irradiation of acute inflammatory conditions must in the first place be easily portable. Since those acutely ill are, at least in private practice, usually confined to bed, it must be possible to bring the lamp to the patient. The small Sollux lamp is therefore constructed as a table outfit (see Fig. 17). The reflector casing and fork bracket are of very light construction; only the detachable foot is made heavy (11 lbs.), for the purpose of stability, but is also easily portable. A hinged joint with brake action at the end of the fork bracket, combined with the axial mounting of the reflector in the fork, enables a range of vertical travel which meets all requirements in practice. All parts are of the same high grade materials as used in the large Sollux lamp, and do not undergo deformation no matter how great the heat developed. At the front end of the reflector funnel is mounted a cork ring as a protection against burns from contact with the hot

F

metal. Behind this ring the red, blue, and daylight filters can be inserted.

The small Sollux lamp is thus specially well suited to all requirements of an apparatus for use at the patient's bedside, but is also equally suited for constant use in one place ; *e.g.*, in the consulting room or out-patients' department.

As well as a table lamp, the Cemach Sollux lamp is also mounted on a light floor stand and on a wall bracket. The stand model is very popular.

6. THE NOLL LARYNX MIRROR.

This device serves to focus the image of the larynx, the irradiation then being left to the patient to carry out for himself.

Fig. 18, below, sufficiently explains the procedure of laryngeal irradiation by manipulation of the small device.

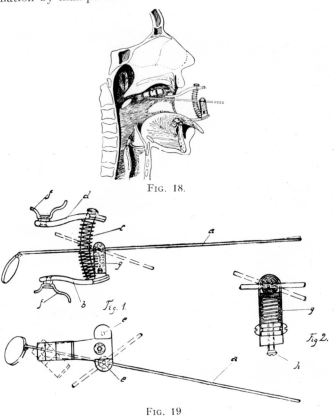

FIG. 18.

FIG. 19

The gag (Fig. 19) consists of a lower arm *b*, on which is fastened a bow-shaped rod *c* of oval section, at the top end of which an upper arm *d* is free to slide up and down, fitting over the rod by an oval aperture. Both arms are pressed apart by a spiral spring acting along the bow-shaped rod. Each arm has a projection by which the arms can be pressed together. The front ends carry the rotatable lip pieces *f*, *f*, which have rubber pads to take the bite.

The lip *e* on the bottom arm carries the pillar in which is mounted the universal joint (Fig. 2, in Fig. 19) for the road on which the throat mirror is mounted. The rod is held between two halves of a ball mounting, pressed together by a spring, with sufficient tension to hold the mirror in any setting yet allowing of full movement in all directions. In use, the gag with mirror in position is introduced into the mouth so that the molars bite on the rubber pads in the lip pieces, the mouth being opened far enough to make the uvula clearly visible when the tongue is extended. If the patient now bites on the gag, his jaws rest on the arms and the instrument remains fixed. If the mouth has to be opened wider, a slight relaxation of the lower jaw effects a wider setting of the gag through the action of the spring.

The mirror, in its holder *g*, is of course always set on the median side of the gag. The apparatus can, however, be used with the base to either the upper or lower jaw, from which it follows that it can be placed in either side of the mouth ; adjustment of the mirror is equally easy in both positions.

7. THE DISTANCE GAUGE.

The effect of ultra-violet radiation diminishes as the square of the distance, so that at two metres distance the effect is approximately only a quarter of that at one metre.

A convenient device for measuring distance, which involves no risk to the burner, is the new Distance Gauge (shown in Fig. 20).

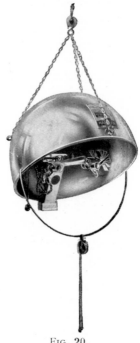

FIG. 20.

It is made in the form of a semicircular frame which pivots from the axis of the burner at each side of the hood, as shown. On the frame is suspended a self-closing metal tape measure, so graduated that the operator can read, at the opening, the distance of the end of the tape from the burner. The range of measurement extends to 130 cms.

8. THE NEON POLE TEST LAMP.

Wrong polarity, with Direct Current outfits, will destroy the burner within a quarter of an hour, entailing expensive repairs. Instances of wrong polarity are of frequent occurrence owing to carelessness when the outfit is installed.

The use of the Neon Pole Test Lamp, either mounted permanently on the hood pins, or used for occasional test by contact with the burner terminals, guards against wrong polarity. The lamp connections are marked in colours, and its terminals made in large and small eyelets, corresponding to the fittings on the quartz burner. The Neon lamp contains two thick interwoven spirals, one with only two turns, the other extending the entire length of the lamp. If the polarity is wrong, the spiral glows along the whole length of the lamp, which is entirely filled with red light. With correct polarity, only the short spiral glows ; *i.e.*, the two turns next the socket, whilst the remainder stays dark.

The device is now available for any direct current supply. It comes into action before the burner is tilted to start ; when the quartz lamp is running, the Pole Test lamp is automatically extinguished.

Part III.

Chapter I.

INTERNAL DISEASES.

Tuberculosis.

THE author's first investigations of the effects produced by the Alpine Sun treatment upon blood pressure were carried out with the patients of a sanatorium for consumptives (*cf. Deutsche Medizinische Wochenschrift*, No. 9, 1911). He also had at the same time opportunities for studying the therapeutic effects of ultra-violet rays on those patients who were in the initial or advanced stages of pulmonary and laryngeal tuberculosis, and whose general condition was weak. After irradiation their condition was greatly improved, and two of them who had been confined to their beds with advanced consumption recovered so far that they could be discharged in considerably improved general condition.

Since then irradiation treatment of tuberculous patients with the quartz or artificial Alpine Sun lamp has been widely practised. The theory is that the irradiations favourably affect the formation of every kind of antigen, more particularly that of the albuminous, and, to a lesser extent, of the fatty antigens to which an important part is ascribed in the cure of tuberculosis. Further, the stimulating effect of the ultra-violet rays on the skin promotes improved circulation, which leads to a favourable reaction upon the tubercular focus, and possibly encourages the excretion of toxin. Since, according to Hoffman, the skin also exercises certain immunizing activities, probably these functions also are stimulated by the action of the ultra-violet rays. In addition to these effects on the tubercular focus and the immunizing processes, the action of the rays upon the patients' general condition is important. Their appetite and sleep are both improved; they feel more fresh and energetic, and their system becomes more able to resist the disease. This statement is not meant to imply that the quartz lamp radiations can cure tuberculosis in all cases. If the organism produces too few protective and curative substances, and if it is flooded by numerous pathological micro-organisms, radiation will be just as useless in preventing death as any other treatment.

PULMONARY AND LARYNGEAL TUBERCULOSIS.

The quartz lamp radiation treatment has proved especially successful during the initial stages of these diseases. The best results are obtained in cases of catarrh and suspicious affections of the apex, and in anæmic subjects with phthisical tendencies, particularly where hereditary predisposition exists. In such cases, the radiation treatment may be designated a specific, with a fair amount of certainty.

Favourable results are also obtained in cases of early hæmorrhage ; and in any case hæmorrhage cannot be regarded as a contra-indication. Numerous observations prove that no further hæmorrhages occur if the radiations are carried out with the requisite care.

Rickman* has arrived at the conclusion that injudicious application of natural insolation, and to a lesser extent of the artificial quartz lamp treatment may frequently cause pulmonary hæmorrhage.

Similarly, ulcerative or fibrotic conditions or cavitation do not constitute contra-indications no matter whether single or double sided, and in artificial pneumothorax treatment radiation has proved a valuable aid to the healing process.

Favourable results have been observed in cases where the diseased foci started from the hilus, and especially in the case of recent tuberculosis of the lymph glands of the hilus. In these instances it is advisable to use a combination of the radiation treatment and deep X-ray therapy, which is quite safe provided that the precautions applicable to the latter are carefully observed.

Fever is not a contra-indication of irradiation treatment, and the assertion that the treatment causes fever has not been confirmed. If an increase of the fever has occasionally been observed after too powerful radiations, this could only have been due to temporary fluctuations of the patient's temperature which have no unfavourable effect upon the course of the disease. Many authors, e.g., Krüger, have reported a gradual fall of temperature subsequent to courses of radiation, which must be interpreted as a favourable symptom. In cases of high temperature David recommends that radiations should be restricted to those hours

*Deutsche Medizinische Wochenschrift, March 3rd, 1922.

during which the patient is free from fever. Above all, he says, they should not be applied immediately the fever subsides, since this period generally coincides with heavy perspiration, which greatly interferes with their curative action.

A common opinion, constantly encountered in literature on actinotherapy, is that it is dangerous to irradiate with a quartz lamp patients with pulmonary tuberculosis, especially in cases where globular and bloody expectoration is present. Menard and Foubert* have investigated the question whether this fear is in fact well founded, or whether the contra-indication may not be ascribed to an accident due to an overdose which produced too much erythema. They have therefore conducted irradiation on cautious lines and avoiding erythema, with gradual increases of dosage, in tubercular cases of all forms and stages. The results have been a uniform improvement in health, accompanied by considerable increase of weight and lowering of temperature, while not one case of hæmorrhage occurred.

The authors therefore came to the conclusion that quartz light irradiation can be employed without disadvantage in all cases of pulmonary tuberculosis, and that only benefit results, provided that irradiation is conducted cautiously and the production of erythema is systematically avoided.

Heusner† has described in detail successes obtained in treating pulmonary tuberculosis. Guttstein‡ has made careful investigations as to the effect of the artificial Alpine Sun treatment upon the lungs, the body as a whole, and the composition of the blood. He reports many instances of improved general condition, and diminution of the cough and expectoration. In a number of cases, fever and bacilli disappeared, patients gained in weight, and increases of hæmoglobin and erythrocytes took place. Frischbier repeats that moist catarrhs dry up and disappear entirely. Bacmeister§ states that he has observed a specific effect of the quartz light on tubercular foci. The favourable action of artificial Alpine Sun irradiation consists primarily in its property of activating

---

*Bull. off. de la Societe Franc d'Electrotherapie, 1925, No. 5.

†Strahlentherapie, vols. vii. and viii.

‡Brauer's Beitrage, vol. xxxv.

§Strahlentherapie, vol. ix.

certain anaphylactic powers of the skin, which are of supreme importance as protective agencies against infection ; further, its power of relieving the congestion of the lungs through its hyperæmic action on the skin, and not least its tonic effect on the heart and the vascular system, thus counteracting the relaxing effect of rest-cures. Hufnagel* states that recent catarrhs of the apex of the lungs are almost invariably improved. Brecke† recommends quartz light wherever it is desired to bring about the disappearance and absorption of pathological products, such as soft granulations and deposits causing thickening of the serous membranes.

Bacmeister points out the advantage of quartz light in pulmonary tuberculosis, in that it can be applied at any time of year or condition of weather, and that by regulation of dosage it is applicable in the weakest and most advanced cases such as could not be exposed to fresh air and sunlight treatment. The general condition, both objective and subjective, is often surprisingly improved, and the continuous hyperæmia of the skin produces a corresponding relief of the pulmonary congestion. This writer recommends the combination of quartz light and X-rays on account of their advantageous effect on the general condition, their general immunizing properties, and their favourable action on the skin, especially in suitable cases of " proliferative " tuberculosis. ‡

The greatest difficulty in treating consumption by the artificial Alpine Sun has hitherto lain in the selection of suitable cases. It has fallen to Fecht§ to overcome this difficulty in the manner outlined below :—

The study of a number of authorities established the following changes in the composition of the blood in respect of the white corpuscles in pulmonary tuberculosis :

1. The leucocyte count is, broadly speaking, normal (leuco-cytosis points to complications).

2. Increase in the neutrophils, with decrease in lymphocytes and eosinophils, is usually evidence of progressive disease.

3. High lymphocyte count, eosinophilia, and decrease in neutrophils points to a favourable course.

*Militärärztliche Zeitschrift, No. 12, 1916.
†Zeitschrift fur Tuberkulose, vol. xxx.
‡Zeitschrift für Tuberkulose, Bad Kösen, 1922.
§Deuts. med. Wochenschrift, 1914, No. 4.

Fecht took into account not only the proportional figures of the total leucocyte count, but also Arneth's more delicate method of diagnosis based on the neutrophil cells, according to which limited polymorphism of the nucleus denotes a younger cell; greater polymorphism, on the other hand, older and more mature leucocytes. Great increase of mononuclear cells is evidence of increased destruction of the mature forms. Arneth classifies the neutrophil forms into five groups, which occur normally in the percentages shown below :—

1st group—mononuclear cells	...	...	about 5%
2nd group—binuclear cells	...	...	about 35%
3rd group—trinuclear cells	...	...	about 41%
4th group—quadrinuclear cells	...	...	about 17%
5th group—quinquenuclear cells	...	...	about 2%

A shift of the normal neutrophil cell count towards the left, *i.e.*, an increase in the number of younger cells with less differentiated nuclei, is often, according to Arneth, an unfavourable sign.

Proceeding from Arneth's principle coupled with the proportional leucocyte values, Fecht formulated the following prognostic table, based on blood tests made before and after three weeks' treatment by quartz light irradiation :—

1. Favourable : Appearance of lymphocytosis with shift of Arneth's values towards the right ; comparative neutropenia. Particularly favourable if accompanied by eosinophilia.

2. Less favourable : Lymphocytosis without a right-hand shift in Arneth's values.

3. Unfavourable : If neither Lymphocytosis nor a right-hand shift in Arneth's values occurs.

4. Bad : Lymphopenia ; neutrophilia ; left-hand shift in Arneth's values.

All sources of error, such as concomitant bronchial asthma, helminthiasis, etc., must be excluded.

On the basis of these findings, quartz lamp irradiation is either continued if successful, or broken off. It is discontinued in all cases coming under groups 3 and 4, which are passed on for sanatorium treatment. If clinical treatment effects a cure, this is usually accompanied by a decrease in the lymphocyte count, while the right-hand shift in Arneth's values remains.

It is urgently necessary to have regard to the clinical manifestations, *i.e.*, the qualitative diagnosis. Aschoff's classification on a pathological-anatomical basis, as codified by Bacmeister, is best suited to this purpose. Bacmeister propounds the following arrangement :—

I.	II.	III.	
Progressive	Cirrhotic ⎫ Proliferative	Closed ⎫ Tuber-	
Stationary	Nodular ⎬	⎬	
Inclined to latency	Broncho-pneumonic ⎫ Exudative /Open	culosis	
Latent	Lobar-pneumonic ⎭	⎭	

IV.

According to area affected.

Right.	Apex (with cavitation)	Left.	Apex (with cavitation)
	Hilus ,,		Hilus ,,
	Upper lobe ,,		Upper lobe ,,
	Middle lobe ,,		Lower lobe ,,
	Lower lobe ,,		

In general, only the forms which are stationary and tending to latency (the cirrhotic, nodular and closed forms) are suited for irradiation, whilst the exudative and open forms, particularly when cavities are present, are unsuitable.

If possible, X-rays should be made use of, and are of valuable assistance.

Fecht employs the following technique : Distance 30 inches ; first radiation 3 minutes each on front and back ; for the second 10 minutes each ; and after this 20 minutes, increasing to 30 minutes, every two or three days.

The combination of Arneth's values and the qualitative leucocyte count gives, after three weeks' irradiation treatment, a definite prognostic basis. In cases of positive or negative discrepancy between general condition and hæmatological findings the further course indicates the prognostic accuracy of this double check. By this means cases suitable for quartz light therapy can be selected and curative treatment continued without irrecoverable loss of time.

It goes without saying that with the quartz light therapy of pulmonary tuberculosis, as in any other morbid condition, dietetic and hygienic measures must not be neglected.

The indications for quartz light irradiation in pulmonary tuberculosis, in so far as intended by some authorities for all forms of this disease, are by many considered too far-reaching, and more precise limitation of dosage is called for. As the main purpose of this introduction is to give a summary of the present state of quartz light therapy, precise directions which shall be valid for each individual case cannot be stated here. It must be left to the practitioner to decide which cases and what dosage he considers suitable for treatment, as may be generally said of any therapeutic measures. Further, quartz light therapy is still too much in the stage of development for a final verdict to be given.

This point of view applies to all diseases discussed in this Introduction.

Dosage : As regards dosage, it has already been pointed out in Part I. of this book that this should not be conducted on set lines, but adapted to individual needs. If the patient is very much run down or suffering from fever, the treatment should start by means of weak radiations as described in Part I. Gradually, however, their intensity should be increased, the distance between the patient and the lamp being reduced, and exposures more and more prolonged. Patients of fairly strong constitution and without fever, in the initial stages of pulmonary or laryngeal tuberculosis, or anæmic tubercular suspects, may be given powerful radiations as soon as their skin has become tanned. General radiation is indicated in all cases, while laryngeal tuberculosis should also be treated by local irradiation. The larynx itself has also been directly radiated, having been made accessible to the rays by means of quartz applicators, but this method would appear applicable in very few cases, owing to the irritability of the parts. Powerful local radiations of those parts of the chest over the tuberculous focus are not advisable if the patient shows any tendency to hæmorrhage ; in such cases general radiation is usually sufficient. Cures cannot, of course, be effected by irradiation in the progressive, exudative and destructive stages of pulmonary or laryngeal tuberculosis, *i.e.*, those cases which are hopeless from the outset.* It may nevertheless be resorted to in such cases, where there are no difficulties of transport or accommodation, as the radiations have a favourable action upon the perspiration, and diminish the feeling of exhaustion. Moreover, if merely the suggestive value of the treatment is taken into account, such unfortunate patients should not be deprived of the faith they may have in radiations as their last hope of

*cf. Kock, Strahlentherapie, vol. xiii., No. 1.

recovery. What is true of many other diseases, is particularly applicable to tuberculosis, that the practitioner is restricted to palliative treatment from which he cannot promise favourable results, if only not to leave the patient without hope. Hence, in such cases irradiation treatment ought to be regarded in the same light as other therapy which is only applied *ut aliquid fiat*. To demand that its use should be restricted to such diseases as promise certain success is not only an unjustifiable interference with the rights of the physician, but is also at variance with his duty to give to his patients any help which he, in his own judgment, considers necessary and suitable.

TUBERCULAR PLEURISY.

The primary forms of this illness are especially suitable subjects for the quartz lamp treatment, both the dry form characterized by fibrous adhesions, and the serous. The absorption of fluid, as a general rule, takes place early, so that it is not advisable to puncture too soon. Long-standing indurative pleurisy is very favourably affected. On the other hand, tubercular empyema is unsuitable for treatment by the quartz lamp. The condition of the lungs must be carefully considered before recourse to radiation treatment.

In addition to the local radiations, general ones are recommended. They must be continued fairly long, and the patient can generally stand them very well, even if they are of great intensity.

TUBERCULOSIS OF THE PERITONEUM AND BOWELS.

These diseases are also suitable for treatment by the quartz lamp, as will be pointed out in detail in the sections of this volume dealing with surgery and children's diseases. The dry form and that accompanied by effusion are best suited for this treatment. No favourable results, however, may be expected in severe cases of ulcerative peritonitis. Laqueur and Lasser-Richter hold that, as regards the prognosis, it is important to note whether a rapid improvement occurs. If no improvement is noticeable after weeks of treatment, these authors are of the opinion that radiations are useless. According to Strehlmann, the quartz lamp treatment surpasses in its effects any other method, and its achievements are especially remarkable where children are concerned. Gassul*

*Prize monograph, published by Gustav Thieme, Leipzig (1921).

states that as a result of the radiations "serous exudates and caseous deposits are either absorbed or changed into fibrous tissue. Anæmia, fever, and diarrhœa disappear simultaneously."

Dosage : If the abdominal walls are very sensitive, the treatment should commence by means of mild local radiations. These should be repeated daily if no erythema is produced. About three days afterwards general radiations may be combined with the local, the whole front of the body being exposed to the lamp mounted vertically above the abdomen. If the radiations are mild at first, and gradually and carefully increased in intensity afterwards, they may be repeated daily or every other day. This is to be continued for weeks or months until a complete cure is achieved.

TUBERCULOSIS OF GLANDS.

The author obtained very successful results in treating this form of tuberculosis by means of the quartz lamp. Large groups of glands near the neck gradually and visibly decreased in size, and the general condition of the patients improved considerably. If the glands have to be removed by operative means, the use of the quartz lamp, subsequent to operation, assists in the process of healing. Favourable results have also been noted in cases of tuberculosis of the hilus and mesenteric glands. Huldschinsky found that the results obtained with children were superior to those obtained with adults. David strongly recommends the use of general radiation if small groups of glands are scattered all over the body. Kovacs failed to see any results in treating inveterate cases of swollen glands and sinuses from glands. Instances of glandular tuberculosis which prove refractory to the artificial Alpine Sun lamp require to be treated by surgical means or by X-rays. The success of the treatment invariably depends on the patient's powers of resistance. These may be raised, by means of brine baths, internal tonics (*e.g.*, cod-liver oil), suitable dieting, and proper care and attention, in addition to irradiation.

Dosage : In addition to general, powerful local radiations should be used, continued for a considerable time. In cases of glandular tuberculosis especially, radiations lasting for hours at a time have proved very successful.

TUBERCULOSIS OF THE KIDNEYS.

Not much need be said here concerning this disease. Rollier

reports good results from Alpine Sunlight treatment, but nothing has been published so far with regard to treatment of this disease by the quartz lamp. It remains to be seen, therefore, whether or not it is a suitable field for this treatment.

NON-TUBERCULAR DISEASES OF THE RESPIRATORY ORGANS.

Cases of acute and chronic bronchitis—especially the latter, and the capillary form of this disease—respond well to quartz lamp treatment. The tendency to cough decreases, and excretion of mucus is facilitated. If emphysema and asthmatic troubles are also present, the latter are relieved, and the patient's general condition is improved. Chronic cases of long standing are not cured by the artificial Alpine Sun treatment, but irradiation may be recommended to give symptomatic relief.

Bronchial asthma cannot be cured by means of irradiation, but the author has observed in various cases that the attacks became less violent and of shorter duration. This observation has been confirmed by Ostermann, of Vienna, and Abels, of Düsseldorf. The author is of opinion that these results cannot be ascribed to any suggestive effects of the ultra-violet rays, but rather to their action on the sympathetic system.

Non-tubercular pleurisy, with and without exudate, is very suitable for treatment by irradiation, satisfactory results being obtained even in cases of empyema. The same holds good for traumatic pleurisy, as was repeatedly observed during the war. Traumatic hæmothorax was absorbed very rapidly by means of ultra-violet radiation. Pleuritic thickening can be removed if fairly long courses of radiation are resorted to. Irradiation with the Sollux lamp is also indicated in pleuritic (non-tubercular) diseases.

The period of convalescence after croupous, bronchial and influenzal pneumonias is shortened by treatment with the quartz lamp. The good results obtained in treating these various diseases are due to the favourable effects of the rays not only upon the local seat of the disease, but also upon the patient's general condition.

Dosage : Apart from local radiation, general light baths are recommended, which should be continued as long and as strong as possible especially in treating thickening of the pleuræ.

INFECTIOUS DISEASES.

A. Chronic Infections.

In treating cases of malaria, Reinhard and May have repeatedly used radiations at brief intervals in order to provoke an attack, and he reports good results by using neo-salvarsan and quinine simultaneously with irradiation. He recommends radiation of the patient on five successive days for one hour each day. Ultra-violet radiation is also suitable to combat the anæmia which almost always occurs with malaria. Cure of malaria by artificial Alpine Sun treatment cannot be expected so long as the parasites are still present.

Breiger has treated syphilis by means of the quartz lamp, artificial Alpine Sun, and reports satisfactory results.* He states that he has cured syphilis exclusively by this means, without using any other treatment. Other writers assert that the quartz lamp treatment achieves no results worth mentioning, that it has even led to an aggravation of the symptoms, and that anæmia due to syphilis is not suitable for this treatment. Kautz, indeed, is of opinion that we are justified in assuming the presence of syphilis, in cases which are of doubtful diagnosis, whenever the radiation method fails, and whenever this failure is accompanied by pain.

On the other hand, Breiger's reports have been confirmed by Hesse. Breiger having always proved a conscientious observer, it would appear advisable to submit his observations to further tests. In cases of malaria and syphilis general radiations on the usual lines are indicated, to be supplemented, as regards the latter disease, by local radiations of the affected parts.

B. Acute Infection.

DIPHTHERIA. Löwenstein has ascertained that the diphtheria toxin is easily destroyed by the quartz light rays. According to experiments carried out by Friedberger the oral cavity of the rabbit is cleared of germs by means of ultra-violet rays. It has been asserted that successful results have been obtained by radiating the germ-carriers, and on the strength of these observations the artificial Alpine Sun lamp has been recommended for purposes of sterilization. So far, however, no absolutely definite

*Münchener Medizinische Wochenschrift, No. 35, 1920.

results can be quoted, and it may perhaps be doubted whether diphtheria is a suitable field for this treatment.

Local radiations of the throat, and general irradiation during the period of convalescence may be worth trying.

INFLUENZA. This complaint is said to have been repeatedly cut short by the quartz lamp method. This is especially the case when the disease is accompanied by catarrh of the upper air passages, as the author can confirm from personal experience. After radiation of the neck and the chest, the tendency to cough is allayed and the excretion of mucus eased.

WHOOPING COUGH. Leopold reports satisfactory results, but Hamburger failed to confirm them. According to Wagner, this complaint is a suitable field for treatment by the artificial Alpine Sun lamp. The author has observed diminution in violence of the attacks subsequent to radiations, but the duration of the illness was not shortened. The results obtained may be ascribed to the fact that the viscid mucus is more easily got rid of. Schotten and Rohr* also report that attacks become less violent and shorter and often cease entirely (*see* section " Diseases of Children ").

Local radiations of the neck and chest, as well as general, are indicated. The latter greatly contribute to an improvement of the patient's general run-down condition.

Acute articular rheumatism and certain other infectious diseases are not suitable for the artificial Alpine Sun lamp, although general radiations during the period of convalescence greatly accelerate the patient's ultimate recovery. They should be weak at first, but slowly increased in intensity from day to day.

DISEASES OF METABOLISM.

Wagner has expressed the view that both the anabolic and catabolic organic processes are affected positively by ultra-violet rays. In this way he accounts for the apparently contradictory fact that, conditions being equal, the adipose tissue sometimes increases, sometimes decreases, as the result of irradiation. He considers that the same is to a certain extent true of the carbo-hydrate purin, albumen, and immunity metabolisms.

In the chapter on " The Effect of General Irradiation on the Organism " (Part I.), some other hypotheses are mentioned which

*Deutsche med. Wochenschrift, 35 (1923) and 45 (1924).

attempt to explain the action of the quartz lamp on the metabolic processes. Since, however, so little is yet known regarding the manner in which these processes actually take place, we must content ourselves with stating the fact that they are stimulated by this treatment. The author has elsewhere given expression to his belief that this stimulating action is due to the effect of the rays upon the functions of the skin. In one paper* he has endeavoured to prove that it is particularly noticeable in the case of those patients suffering from gout with hereditary or acquired dryness of the skin. Such skin is limited in perspiring capacity and does not excrete large quantities of liquid or solid substances. The stimulating action of quartz lamp rays shows improvement in these respects, thus acting as an antidote to the accumulation of uric acid in the body. The uric acid, of course, originates in consequence of certain other organic processes, and must be treated in the first place by suitable dieting, but if we are in a position to promote its discharge from the body, much is gained. Experience has shown that any kind of stimulation of the activities of the skin, e.g., by means of baths, in the case of gout, is of benefit, even if no very obvious variation from the normal condition and functions of the skin are noticeable. The quartz lamp radiations supply a specific means of stimulating and improving the activity of the skin, and therefore of combating gout and gouty disposition, especially in the case of irregular uric acid metabolism due to deficient functions of the skin. According to the research work of H. Königsfeld (see pp. 23-24), it increases the entire metabolism, above all the albumin metabolism.

The favourable effect of the rays upon patients suffering from diabetes, observed by Lampé, may presumably be ascribed to the same causes, since such subjects generally suffer from dry skin and deficient action of the skin.

The successful results obtained in the treatment of obesity by quartz lamp irradiation have been ascribed by Wagner to stimulation of the assimilatory processes. In such cases, particularly those suffering from anæmia, fatty degeneration, or cardiac weakness, the tonic action of the radiations is also beneficial.

The cure of a case of diabetes insipidus by means of artificial

---

* " Über Disposition und Behandlung der Gicht mit ultravioletten Licht," published in vol. xvi. (1912) of the *Zeitschrift für Physikalische und Diätetische Therapie.*

Alpine Sun treatment, reported by the author in No. 43 of the Deutsche Medizinische Wochenschrift (1911), is by many ascribed to the effect of irradiation upon the metabolism. The author refrained in his paper from attempting to account for this cure, but rather inclines to the view that this was a case of resolution of stasis accompanied by traces of earlier suppuration of the middle ear, operatively treated, the resulting nervous tensions from which caused dryness of the mouth and polydipsia, which, in its turn, caused polyuria. At any rate, the polydipsia did not disappear until the mouth ceased to be dry.

Arteriosclerosis—which must also be regarded as primarily a disturbance of the metabolic functions of the circulatory system and nerve centres, in which uric acid metabolism plays a part—is also favourably affected by the quartz lamp treatment. Long-standing cases, with hardened arteries and serious heart trouble, are not fit subjects for treatment, but the initial stages of the disease are very favourably affected by irradiation. The circulation improves considerably, noises in the head and attacks of dizziness disappear, and the patient's general condition is improved. The blood pressure is reduced, and an improvement effected in the patient's appetite, sleep, and general fitness.

In dealing with metabolic diseases of all kinds, dietetic treatment must not be neglected.

General radiations of the usual type are indicated. They should be continued for a long time, and become gradually more and more powerful.

According to Pincussen's researches,* sensitizers, particularly fluorescent dyes and eosin above all, intensify the action of quartz light irradiation on the metabolism of purins, carbohydrates and albumin, after preliminary treatment with potassium iodide ; a fact of which therapeutic use may be made. In many cases of gout, even of the so-called atypical form, such treatment led to results which were successful, both objectively and subjectively regarded. The same was true of diabetes, treated in combination with dietetic measures. The therapeutic procedure for treating gout and diabetes consists in the administration of 0.25 to 0.5 eosin, internally, about one hour before the ultra-violet irradiation. According to experiments on veterinary and human subjects, uric acid disappears under this treatment, and in diabetes this procedure

*Strahlentherapie, 17 (1924).

leads to favourable results, although they are sometimes slow. Acidosis also is usually abated by this means.

CHRONIC ARTICULAR RHEUMATISM.

As regards the chronic secondary forms, periarthritis destruens, and osteoarthritis deformans (Umber), radiation treatment has little direct influence on the local seat of the disease. Since, however, they are mostly accompanied by anæmia and general weakness, treatment by the artificial Alpine Sun may improve the patient's general condition materially. General radiation over a long period should be employed in such cases. Kliashkin,* when treating polyarthritis with quartz light, particularly fresh cases, obtained 80% cures. In sciatica, 30% cures, 60% improvement, and in only 10% of cases no change. In neuritis, only a certain degree of improvement was recorded, *i.e.*, diminution of pain in the nerve stem when subjected to pressure, and of the disturbances of sensitivity.

Reh† treated the following conditions with the artificial light radiations :—

1. Diseases of the capsular ligament, ligaments, and adjacent muscles and sinews.

2. Synovial diseases with only slight involvement of the neighbouring joint surfaces.

3. Diseases with extensive destruction of the adjacent smooth surfaces, *e.g.*, in the joints.

The results were as follows :—

1. Both acute and long-standing cases were cured without exception, in very short time, and no relapses occurred.

2. Cure resulted after many irradiations, but relapses occurred when treatment was not repeated about eight times.

3. Irradiation resulted in alleviation of pain, after a few hours of increased sensitivity. Neither cure nor permanent decrease of pain could be achieved.

Further, Reh successfully treated various forms of neuralgia (particularly sciatica), using ordinary dosage. His view is that neuralgias are not the effects of cold alone, but are infections,

*Kazan Med. Weekly, 1924, No. 7.
†Strahlentherapie, 14 (1922).

mostly from bacteria existing in the body, externally activated by the action of cold. The first improvement appears very probably due to increased supply of anti-toxins at the time of treatment, and the permanent result to lasting improvement in the vascular conditions.

Reh speaks of a " pain-dose " and a " curative dose." The latter are three or four times the former. The degree of dosage necessary is dependent on the duration of the process, and its extent. Fresh cases all respond in a short time and result in cures, long-standing cases show only a slight improvement, particularly alleviation of pain.

MUSCULAR RHEUMATISM.

The acute types of this disease are very suitable for artificial Alpine Sun treatment. In many instances, the pain can be alleviated, and movement improved by means of one single powerful local radiation. Radiation may be continued until pronounced reddening of the skin, or even blisters, are produced ; mild ointment (e.g., Hanoviol Healing Ointment) soon removes any ill effects.

The chronic types of this disease also respond well to the radiation treatment. As but little is known concerning them, and their cure is frequently complicated by difficulties, we are restricted to symptomatic treatment. Intensive local radiations repeated when the skin erythema has subsided, are of great benefit, as are also heat radiations with the Sollux lamp, which can be combined with the artificial Alpine Sun treatment. The first session, in the treatment of both the acute and chronic forms, should last from ten to fifteen minutes.

DISEASES OF THE NERVOUS SYSTEM.

Brustein* reported successful results in treating sciatica, and neuralgia of the trigeminus, occipitalis, brachialis, and intercostalis by means of quartz light radiation, and his statements have subsequently been corroborated by Kalle, Sokolow, and others. It has also proved helpful in cases of neurosis of the heart, neurasthenia, hysteria, and chorea, and the author of this volume has also observed beneficial results in certain cases of

*Writing in vol. xiii., No. 9, of the *Zeitschrift für Physikalische und Diätetische Therapie* (1909/10).

enuresis with patients highly sensitive to the effects of cold. Wagner's successes with epileptic patients have been referred to in Part I.* (*cf.* the chapter on the action of general radiations on the organism).

Various writers have ascribed these successful results in treating nervous disorders, to suggestion. A certain suggestive influence is probable with artificial Alpine Sun treatment, as with any other therapeutic remedy, but the very fact that erythema is caused by the ultra-violet rays is a sure sign that suggestion does not account for all its effects. It is much more probable that the successful results are due to the action of the rays on the metabolic functions and the circulatory system, and that their direct effect on the sympathetic system plays a considerable part. Lazarus has shown that angio-neurotic conditions, arteriospastic phenomena, and paræsthesia due to vasomotor disturbances are favourably affected by the artificial Alpine Sun treatment, and Königsfeld, in his valuable paper,† has proved its incontestable influence on the metabolic functions.

In cases of acute neuralgia, one single powerful local radiation is often sufficient to stop the pain. In chronic cases, especially with patients whose skin is extremely sensitive, a start should be made with weak local radiations. As the patient's entire nervous system is usually highly sensitive, these local radiations should be supplemented by general ones, weak at first, and cautiously increased later.

Cases of neurosis of the heart, neurasthenia, hysteria, chorea, enuresis, and epilepsy should be treated only by general radiation. These should be adapted to the sensibility of the patient's skin and should generally be weak at first. In addition, however, there are cases with arteriospastic phenomena which react with difficulty to ultra-violet rays. In these instances even the first radiation may be powerful (about ten minutes' exposure at a distance of 24 to 28 inches). The next treatment should not be given until after the disappearance of the erythema. In order to avoid too long intervals between the various radiations, it is advisable to radiate during one sitting the front and at the next sitting the back of the body.

*cf. *Zeitschrift für Physikalische und Diätetische Therapie*, vol. xix., 1915.

†*Zeitschrift für Klinische Medizin*, vol. xci., Nos. 3 to 6.

DISEASES OF THE CIRCULATORY SYSTEM.

Since, as the author has shown, the application of the artificial Alpine Sun treatment reduces the blood pressure (as has been confirmed by Lenkei, Lindhard, Lampé, and Strassner), cases of increased blood pressure are suitable for radiation therapy. Serious cases of arteriosclerosis combined with a very high blood pressure do not lend themselves to this treatment, as has already been pointed out in the section on metabolic diseases. Menzer and Thedering, even, deprecate its application in such instances. It is, however, beneficial in the initial stages of arteriosclerosis.

Among the diseases of the heart, weakness due to serious illness or to over-exertion, and with accompanying secondary anæmia, are specially suitable for the artificial Alpine Sun treatment. Its application relieves the heart, so that the patient's breathing becomes deeper and slower, while sleep also improves. No results are to be expected from it in cases of valvular defects and severe compensatory disturbances, although less serious cases of this kind are favourably affected.

Dosage : Only general irradiation should be applied. It should be weak at first (three to five minutes' exposure at a distance of 40 inches from the patient) and gradually increased in intensity.

ANAEMIA AND CHLOROSIS.

Anæmias following severe loss of blood, serious illness, and accompanying exhaustion or other cachexia are very suitable for the artificial Alpine Sun treatment. The radiations promote the formation of erythrocytes and hæmoglobin. Although the investigations of Hansen, Berner, Bardenheuer, and Traugott have failed to give an exact explanation of these biological effects, practical experience has shown that these anæmic conditions are very favourably affected by the artificial Alpine Sun treatment, and that they speedily improve.

In cases of pernicious anæmia and anæmia due to tumours, irradiation should not be applied. Many instances of improvement have been recorded, but the fundamental complaint cannot be influenced by the rays.

Chlorosis responds very favourably to the artificial Alpine Sun treatment. The successful results are mainly due to the stimulating effect of the radiations upon the metabolism. In cases which are accompanied by weakness of the cardiac muscle and functional murmurs, their strengthening effect on the heart also contributes greatly towards recovery.

Berner and others have ascertained that the skin of patients suffering from anæmia or chlorosis often shows very slight pigmentation as a result of radiation, from reasons connected with the general condition of the skin in individual cases (*cf.* the chapter on pigmentation in Part I.). As a rule, sufferers from malnutrition rapidly gain in weight, whereas those abnormally adipose through sluggish metabolism frequently lose weight owing to the enhanced activity of combustion. The same observation has also been made with patients whose tissues contained an excessive amount of water. In such instances the diuresis is increased, and the tissues drained of excessive water.

Dosage : Only general radiation is needed. It should be weak at first, and gradually be made more powerful.

LEUCAEMIA.

The application of the quartz lamp treatment to this disease is limited to the improvement of the injured erythroblastic mechanism which may result. Berner[*] has proved that the radiations affect the leucocytes. The leucocyte count, particularly as regards the polynuclear cells, decreases, but the lymphocytes remain unchanged, or even increase slightly. The neutrophil leucocytosis which Walscheff has shown to result from local radiation, depending in amount on the duration of the radiation and the area radiated, has scarcely any importance with respect to leucæmia as a general condition, although this local phenomenon probably accounts for the favourable effect of irradiation on furuncles, etc. The dosage is the same as for anæmia.

KIDNEY DISEASE.

David takes the view that artificial Alpine Sun treatment is of use in kidney troubles, but only in cases where anæmia has developed, or if the activity of the patient's skin requires stimulation. Hence, cases of nephrosis or nephritis, accompanied by extensive retention of nitrogen residue or indican, would be suitable subjects.

Ebel has obtained successful results in cases of kidney disease and Wagner confirms this observation, mentioning reduction of

[*]*Strahlentherapie*, No. 9, 11, 1914.

the blood pressure, relief of heart strain, and stimulation of diuresis as among the results obtained.

Thedering, on the other hand, does not recommend the treatment for these diseases.

Considering the mutual interdependence existing between the functions of the heart, the skin, and the kidneys, it would seem reasonable to assume that the action of artificial Alpine Sun treatment on the skin and the heart should also extend to the activities of the kidneys. No exact investigations of this question have been made so far, but the experience gained in practice has shown that radiations favourably affect the circulation and diuresis. In cases of contracted kidney, the author has observed that two or three irradiations a week applied for a period of four weeks, lasting from eight to twenty minutes each time at a distance of 20 inches, reduce the blood pressure, relieve the headache, and improve both the patient's sleep and his general condition. If the skin is highly sensitive to the light, the radiations should be weak at first and gradually increased in intensity.

STOMACH AND BOWEL DISEASES.

Wagner observed that in these diseases irradiation led to improvement of appetite and increase of weight. Ostermann achieved satisfactory results in cases of hyper-secretion of the stomach, without applying any other remedy. Delacheux states that he brought about improvements in cases of spastic and hyper-secretory diseases.

The author regards powerful local radiations as effective in cases of atony of the stomach and intestines. The strong epidermal irritation increases the functional activity of these organs. As already mentioned in the section dealing with anæmia, general radiation has also proved useful in cases of secondary anæmia due to chronic stomach and bowel troubles, e.g., ulcers of the stomach and the duodenum.

In this connection it should be stated that successful results have also been observed in diseases of the liver, and pancreatic deficiency (cf. Wagner, Herzing, and the author). Enlargement of the liver caused by passive congestion is particularly suitable for treatment, but malignant diseases are not affected. The explanation of the successes obtained is that the powerful irritation of the skin stimulates the activities of the organs in question, and that congestion is removed.

GOITRE.

Langemak* recommends the use of quartz light irradiation in cases of small and infantile goitre ; also in cases with larger tumour, particularly where parenchymatous and morbid colloidal changes were present, he obtained successful results unaccompanied by injury, provided that the case was not complicated by irregularity or acceleration of the heart's action. It is, however, essential to watch the urine strictly and to keep the case under supervision. Treatment is given on the average three times weekly for ten minutes at a distance of 20 inches, after the burner has been allowed three to five minutes for starting.

The writer's technique is to prolong the irradiation period to twenty or thirty minutes, and he has obtained successful results after about fifteen exposures. Local irradiations are indicated, which may be assisted by general light baths.

In exophthalmic goitre, irradiation is indicated for the relief of pain, and is as a rule well tolerated. Cure of the condition cannot be achieved by this means.

Kliatshkin† reports, regarding the treatment of exophthalmic goitre with quartz light, that he observed diminution of the thyroid, abatement of tachycardia, of hyperhidrosis, and of tremor. The patients were subjectively better, were more tranquil, and the pulse, heart's action, and respiration improved. Insomnia was also favourably affected by quartz lamp treatment.

CONVALESCENCE.

It was observed, especially during the war, that patients recovered with striking rapidity after quartz light treatment. Jesionek, in a lecture at the Post-graduate Medical Course at Kreuznach in May, 1925, explains this as follows :—Ultra-violet rays stimulate the basal cells of the epidermis, not only in their pigment bearing but in their germinative and keratoplastic capacity. The light which is absorbed is transformed not only into pigment but also, so to speak, into horny substance. The epidermis develops to its full capacity under this light action on the basal cells, and becomes

---

*Deutsche Zeitschrift f. Chir., vol. clxxvii.

†Kasan med. Zeitschrift, 1924, No. 7.

thicker. The stratum corneum of the irradiated epidermis is stronger and more resistant than of the non-irradiated. In many morbid affections affecting the keratin forming process, light is able to restore the physiological action. To this property of the basal cells is due the body's protection by the epidermis against all external forces, and this protective effect is the more complete since the horny substance contains an admixture of certain fatty and oily matters, the so-called " horn fat," the formation of which proceeds *pari passu* with the process of keratization. In this manner light is able to impart the properties of a protective organ to the epidermis.

The basal cells, which are endowed with a high degree of vitality, also give out metabolic products of themselves and start processes which affect the entire organism, since their chemical products are given out into the circulation. The cutaneous vascular system also reacts to the action of light, either by means of the basal cells (Jesionek's view) or, as others hold, by direct action on the vessel walls. This action of ultra-violet light is assisted by the visible rays which have a thermic action and penetrate deeper into the tissues.

The action of light further results in the formation of new connective tissue cells as a consequence of improved nutrition, and Rothmann holds that more albumin constituents, tyrosin and phenylalanin, pass from the basal cells into the blood circulation. In the cells an oxidizing ferment changes the chromogenic substances into melanin. Jesionek regards the melanin granules as an intermediate stage in the production of substances which are formed by the basal cells and which carry the light energy into the body economy ; *i.e.*, absorption of light by the skin sets up action due to light in the blood, the bones, the lungs, etc. Diminution of blood pressure and lowering of the blood sugar content proceed *pari passu* with this. This action fits in with the idea of hypertonicity of the sympathetic nervous system, and in Rothmann's view is due to a primary paresis of the sympathetic nerve-endings in the skin, caused by light. In Jesionek's view, the terminals of the sympathetic nervous system are located in the nuclei of the basal cells of the epidermis, so that the dual result of light absorption by the nucleus is due on the one hand to transformation of the chromogenic substance into melanin, on the other to paresis of the sympathetic nerve terminals.

As a result of the functional depression of the sympathetic, the internal organs receive a more abundant supply of blood, a fact of great importance in cases of weakness, enfeeblement, and convalescence.   Other effects of the sympathetic hypotonicity are the relative lymphocytoses, slight increase of the mononuclear cells, and eosinophilia ; and also, according to Königsfeld, the definite effect on the leucocyte count observed after irradiation.

Of greater practical importance is the increase of blood-calcium content due to light action, which persists long after irradiation. This plays an important part not only in tuberculosis and rickets, but also in convalescence.

The action of light on metabolism as a whole is also particularly marked in the increase of weight during convalescence, frequently astonishing in its amount, which occurs even when the diet is comparatively poor in nitrogenous content owing to better assimilation of the proteins.   Königsfeld has shown that with the artificial Alpine Sun irradiation there is at first increased nitrogen metabolism, greater excretion of nitrogen and of phosphorus, sulphur and common salt, but that the increased excretion is succeeded after a few days by increased nitrogen retention.   According to Königsfeld irradiation stimulates the appetite, and the increased food intake in turn assists the positive albumin formation caused by light.   Wiener made similar observations.   According to him, diseases accompanied by loss of albumin respond markedly to irradiation ; tuberculosis, pernicious anæmia, exophthalmic goitre, etc.

" The irradiated skin is of a warmer red and brown tone, full and thick, glossy, taut, firm, resilient, elastic, soft, flexible, and feels like velvet.   It has a dull gloss through the presence of small yet adequate amounts of that ' horn fat ' which is the property of the well-developed *stratum corneum*.   It is not cold and dry to the touch, but rather marked by a certain richness and moisture, the result of normal action of the fatty sulphuric acid function of the sebaceous glands, and is also covered with a fine down of woolly hair on the appropriate parts of the body.

" The skin of diseased and convalescent subjects, especially under the action of clothing which cuts off light, is marble white or pale as a corpse, without blood or pigment ; thin, limp and lax, cold, dry, scaly, without richness or gloss.   Microscopic investigations show that the epidermis, with its basal cells poor or lacking in pigment, is thin and deficient in cells. The individual layers of the epidermis and the various layers of the connective tissue are poorly developed, the arterial blood vessels are narrow and scanty, whilst the venous blood vessels are dilated ; the moisture content of the connective tissue and outer skin is deficient."

In this manner Jesionek lays down " that the therapy for convalescence should aim at restoring to the skin its natural constitution by means of artificial Alpine Sun irradiation ; *i.e.,* to expose the skin to that vital stimulus which is indeed able to promote its specific functions, particularly those of the basal cells, and thereby to confer valuable benefits on the entire organism."

———

SUMMARY.

Artificial Alpine Sun treatment has proved successful in the case of the following internal diseases :—

Incipient pulmonary and laryngeal tuberculosis (catarrhs of the apex and suspicious apical affections), also the advanced forms, and those kinds which originate with the hilus (glandular tuberculosis).

Tubercular pleurisy.

Tuberculosis of the peritoneum and bowels, especially the dry and serous forms.

Glandular tuberculosis.

Acute and chronic bronchitis.

Bronchial asthma.

Non-tubercular pleurisy and thickening of the pleuræ.

Traumatic hæmothorax.

Convalescence after pneumonia.

Malarial anæmia.

Syphilis.

Influenza.

Metabolic diseases (gout, diabetes, incipient arteriosclerosis).

Muscular rheumatism.

Diseases of the nervous system (neuralgia, neurosis of the heart, neurasthenia, hysteria, chorea, enuresis, epilepsy).

Cardiac weakness, and minor compensatory disturbances.

Anæmia and chlorosis.

Stomach and bowel troubles (enlargement of the liver from congestion and pancreatic deficiency).

Goitre (but not exophthalmic goitre).

Convalescence.

Whooping cough.

In the following diseases successful results have not yet been definitely established :—

Diphtheria.

Kidney diseases.

Leucæmia.

Contra-indications :—

Tubercular empyema.

Severe ulcerous peritonitis.

Acute articular rheumatism.

Valvular disease of the heart, with serious disturbances of compensation.

Severe arteriosclerosis.

Pernicious and tumorous anæmias.

CHAPTER II.

SURGERY.

THIS chapter is based on the clinical portion of " Die Queck-silberdampf-Quarzlampe ' Kunstliche Hohensonne,' "* by Dr. Werner Budde, of the Surgical Clinic, University of Halle, by permission of the author.

A. NON-SPECIFIC DISEASES AND INFECTED WOUNDS.

Surgical, aseptic operation wounds are not, as a rule, indications for irradiation treatment ; only for cosmetic reasons has the artificial Alpine Sun occasionally been used. In plastic operations on the face Budde has made frequent but cautious use of local irradiation. Acceleration of the healing process through active vascularization, and a favourable effect on the nutrition of many of the skin flaps with narrow attachments was often recognizable.

The fact that he had to deal with injuries under non-aseptic conditions was partly responsible for inducing him to resort to artificial Alpine Sun treatment. Thus, inflammatory phenomena subsequent to plastic work by means of skin flaps (*e.g.*, when closing penetrating sinuses) frequently subsided.

Virchow's observation that scars healing under the influence of light are of particular fineness has been confirmed by the use of ultra-violet rays (compare Kromayer, Becker, etc.). Keloids are stated to be favourably affected and softened by means of powerful local radiation, and the stimulating effect of the treatment on the growth of epithelium has occasioned its application to sensitive scars for the purpose of hardening them off.

More important now, however, in aseptic surgery is the use of irradiation in gaping wounds, and particularly when loss of skin has occurred ; this application gained prominence in the treatment of casualties during the war. The artificial Alpine Sun, owing to its undoubted effectiveness, has gained numerous friends on this account, but it would be wrong to over-estimate its achievements by expecting too much from it.

The effect of irradiation depends, in the first place, upon the

---

*Published as vol. xiii. of *Ergebnisse der Chirugie.*

time of its application. It makes all the difference whether we irradiate a recent wound, still fighting against necrosis, foreign bodies and bacilli; or whether the struggle is over, so that the process of healing, accompanied by the formation of granulations and epithelium, is proceeding to a normal conclusion.

In the case of clean flat injuries to fleshy parts of the body, caused by the violent action of some blunt instrument, and associated with serious damage and destruction to the surrounding tissues, the quartz lamp treatment is beneficial during the former phase; and the same holds good if destruction of the tissue has been caused by serious primary infection. The action of the rays in such cases is due to their sero-tactic and hyperæmia-producing qualities. Secretion is promoted, so that the whole area affected by the injury is pervaded by the germicidal substances and anti-toxins contained in the serum. The hyperæmia increases the resisting powers of the organism against the hæmorrhagic and septic serous infiltrations. The results are deodorization, accelerated demarcation, and the elimination of the necrotic tissue; and these are often obtained in a remarkably short time if the artificial Alpine Sun is used. Subjective relief from the nervous tension of the inflammation accompanies the cleansing of the wound.

Radiation should be commenced with the artificial Alpine Sun at 20 inches distance, for exposures of ten to twenty minutes, the parts surrounding the wound being covered. As a rule, a few sessions are sufficient.

The beneficial effects of artificial Alpine Sun treatment in paronychia, boils, and carbuncles may be similarly explained.

In the case of cleansed, well-granulating wounds only such mild radiations as increase the biological power of reaction of the cells without injuring them, may be expected to promote the process of healing. In these instances, therefore, cautious dosage is advisable, *i.e.*, the first few sessions should last from five to ten minutes only with the lamp at 40 inches distance.

On the other hand, if the process of healing is slow, especially if torpid and soft granulations are present, more powerful stimulation by the artificial Alpine Sun should be aimed at. Intense local radiations, for instance, in the case of *ulcus cruris* act in the same way as any other irritant. The parts surrounding the ulcer must be covered. Breiger has drawn attention to the healing of secondary syphilitic ulcers.

Tomasone,* of the Dermo-Syphilopathic Clinic of the Royal University of Naples, irradiated chancre-buboes with quartz light (five to fifteen minutes at 70-40 cms. distance), and found that ultra-violet rays had a decidedly favourable action on this kind of bubo at any stage, both after incision and drainage and also without incision. The formation of scars was obviated. Cure takes place after one or at most two weeks, using daily irradiation. Non-infective chancres also are assisted by ultra-violet treatment without other therapeutic measures.

Dietz, of Bromberg, cured a case of serpiginous *ulcus molle,* which resisted the usual therapeutic methods, within a week by artificial Alpine Sun treatment. He began with exposures of five minutes at 10 inches distance, and irradiated daily until healing occurred. Similar good results were obtained in further cases. He upholds the treatment even as a method of differential diagnosis, since a syphilitic ulcer will respond only with extreme slowness to irradiation, while a soft chancre soon displays healing tendencies.

Hirsch, of Chicago, cured epididymitis by quartz light and heat ray treatment.

Similar conditions obtain in the case of wounds, complicated by other injuries, especially if the treatment (immobilization) admits of it ; the radiations may be used with advantage during the first stage as an additional stimulation, and the instructions given for the treatment of flesh wounds apply here also. Kovacs, Breiger, Kriser, Jesionek and other authors have observed that radiation facilitates the elimination of foreign bodies, and accelerates the sequestration of decomposing bone particles.

If wounds of any kind are accompanied by organic disease such as tuberculosis or syphilis, the artificial Alpine Sun treatment has proved beneficial not only for the patient's general condition, but also for the healing of the wound and the formation of scar-tissue. Hence, general radiations for strengthening the exhausted functions are especially recommended.

Prominence has recently been given to the artificial Alpine Sun irradiation of recent operation wounds. Healing is thereby accelerated, with good cicatrization ; and provided that radiations are not only local, but also general, they assist convalescence.

*Riforma Medica, 1925, No. 14.

They may be begun as early as the second or third day after the operation, and administered daily, provided that a strong erythema is avoided. It is advisable to begin with mild radiations (five minutes' exposure ; 32 to 40 inches) and to increase with caution.

The effect of artificial Alpine Sun treatment upon the vascular system has led to its successful use in cases of nutritional disturbances, such as those caused by vascular spasm and arteriosclerosis, and of senile gangrene* ; and further, for the restoration of normal circulation, and the acceleration of demarcation in cases of frostbite, burns, and chemical burns. According to Wagner, treatment of frostbite is more effective if combined with incisions and hot air treatment.

Wounds infected with *bacillus pyocyaneus*, especially when of a superficial character, show good results under artificial Alpine Sun treatment.† The irradiations should be of medium strength, beginning with five to ten minutes at 40 inches distance ; after a few sessions, the bluish pus disappears altogether.

Several authors, *e.g.*, Beck, Carl, Capelle, and Klapp, have warmly recommended the artificial Alpine Sun in the treatment of erysipelas, although others have advised against undue optimism. The contradictory opinions expressed are probably due to the great diversity in the course of this disease with different individuals. Melin, of Stockholm, surrounded the erysipelatous area with a reddened and oedematous zone in the healthy skin, an inch in width, by means of quartz light, giving five minutes' irradiation at 20 cm. distance, and was thereby enabled to limit the erysipelas and to achieve a rapid cure. If the irradiation is sufficiently powerful, a single treatment suffices.

Mayer,‡ of Werden, used irradiation in two cases of spreading erysipelas, from the first day for two minutes at 80 cms. distance, on the second for three minutes at 60 cms., then four minutes at 50 cms., so increasing gradually by three minutes up to fifteen minutes at 50 cms. distance, both on the front and back of the body. The pyrexia abated gradually from one session to the next, the progress of the erysipelas was checked, and the disease slowly abated. After about six treatments the cases were cured.

*Kriser.

†*Koch and Baeumer, Jesionek, Eisenbach.*

‡*Zeitschrift für Arztl. Fortbildung*, 1924, No. 4.

E. v. Redwitz* applied the artificial Alpine Sun in some chronic cases of erysipeloid, and came to the view that this treatment greatly assists the usual therapeutic measures.

According to Bange† the good results achieved with quartz light in erysipelas are based on the production of a local hyperæmia.

Brünauer‡ assumes that the morbid processes obtaining in the inflamed area are restricted and weakened under the action of the artificial Alpine Sun, so that conditions are thereby achieved which are less favourable to the streptococci. He irradiated chiefly the margins of the diseased area.

Tetanus was first treated successfully with the artificial Alpine Sun by Siemon, Jesionek, Jakobstal, and Tamm. According to Jesionek, the action of light in increasing oxygen metabolism and intensifying phagocytic action is accompanied by a complementary reaction at the focus of infection which he ascribes to the saturation of the wound with serum. This author, among others, recommends very powerful local radiations at the beginning of treatment (from half-an-hour to five hours, and in most instances use of the Uviol blue filter is necessary).

In cases of what is called " latent infection "—which has acquired a certain importance as regards war surgery—artificial Alpine Sun treatment is advantageous owing to its hyperæmia-producing properties and the resultant softening of the scars.

Gotthardt,§ among others, cured X-ray ulcers with quartz light, which can be used at any stage of the ulceration.

The action of the artificial Alpine Sun in promoting vascularization accelerates the resorption of extravasated blood and fluid in the body cavities. Kapp accounts for this action on the assumption that the induced hyperæmia of the skin from physical stimulation causes analogous phenomena in the blood vessels of the intestines. Hufnagel and Bogdanik have reported isolated instances of beneficial effects from radiation, applied to the treatment of non-specific exudates, such as *empyema pleurae*.

Mention may here be made of an article by Prof. Eduardo Semprun, of Madrid, in the *Karlsbader ärztl. Vorträgen* for 1922, on the future treatment of carcinoma. He observed that the

*Münch. Med. Wochenschrift, 1924, No. 25.

†*Arch. für Klin. Chirug.*, vol. cxxvii., 1923.

‡*Med. Klinik*, No. 29, 1924.

§*Fortschritte auf dem Gebiete der Röntgenstrahlen*, vol. xxx., No. 6, 1922.

resistance of neoplastic cells is not changed in the slightest degree when they are injected into the living plasma, after exposure to X and radium radiations. On the other hand, their resistance is totally destroyed by irradiation with ultra-violet rays from the artificial Alpine Sun. They then disappear in the living plasma like any other cell. On this observation he has based the following treatment of carcinoma, which he terms " concealed luminescence ":—The patient is injected daily with 20 grammes of a physiological anæsthetizing serum and 2 grammes of concentrated solution of quinine with eosin and fluorescin which has been exposed for two hours to ultra-violet rays from the quartz lamp. Nothing could be gathered concerning the results of his treatment and no reports by other practitioners are available.

B. Tuberculosis.

The artificial Alpine Sun treatment of certain cases of organic tuberculosis, with which the surgeon is often confronted, differs in nothing from that of tuberculosis of the bones, joints, and the deeper seated tissues ; and these forms are therefore here included under the heading " Surgical Tuberculosis."

Cases of *peritonitis tuberculosa* were treated at the surgical clinic of Halle University in 1918, with the following results :—

	Cured.		Greatly improved.		Unaffected.		Died.		Total.
	(a)	(b)	(a)	(b)	(a)	(b)	(a)	(b)	
(1) Not radiated ...	–	–	4	4	1	–	–	–	5
(2) Inadequately radiated	–	–	4	1	9	1	2	–	15
(3) Adequately radiated	2	–	10	3	–	–	2	1	14
Total ...	2	–	18	8	10	1	4	1	34

N.B.—Column (a) denotes the total number of cases concerned.
Column (b) denotes the number of those operated upon.

In every instance general radiations were employed, their intensity being cautiously increased. The term " inadequate " in the above table denotes a number of treatments under 30, from 10 to 15 radiations being as a rule necessary to establish tolerance to exposures of one hour each. Of the 20 patients who were not radiated, or not adequately radiated, 8 showed considerable improvement, including 5 operated cases ; no effect was produced in 10 cases, including 1 patient who was also operated upon. The two patients who died were children suffering from the malignant septic ulcerative type of *peritonitis tuberculosa*, who were hopeless cases when they entered the clinic. The other patients, on the whole, were suffering from the less severe forms of the disease, mostly from serous *peritonitis tuberculosa*. Those who were adequately radiated, *i.e.*, who received 30-200 or more treatments, included two (serous form) who left the clinic completely cured after having been radiated for about a year without having undergone operative or any other important treatment. Of the remaining twelve, 10 were considerably improved ; treatment was in many cases of a combined form and included three operations, also deep X-ray action, and hot-air treatment, natural sunlight, and open-air baths. Two children with severe forms of the disease died, one a long time after laparotomy. The tendency towards healing apparent under the third heading of the table is unmistakable when the treatment is extended over three months or more ; but the net result must be evaluated with regard to every therapeutic factor employed. The same holds good for all other forms of tuberculosis, so that statistics of results of artificial Alpine Sun treatment itself cannot be obtained from the tables.

According to König's experience with a large number of surgical tuberculosis patients, covering a period of eighteen months, the number of major operations necessary before the introduction of the artificial Alpine Sun treatment was 21 out of a total of 79 patients, but diminished to 4 out of a total of 85 cases afterwards. In the surgical clinic of Halle University, the corresponding figures were 67 cases of tuberculosis of large joints and spinal caries with 8 major operations (11·9%) prior to the introduction of the quartz lamp treatment (and to the war), as against 204 such cases and 18 operations (8·7%) in 1918 These results indicate progressive improvement of the conservative methods.

It is difficult to say how far this improvement is due to the direct and indirect effects of artificial Alpine Sun treatment. Jesionek and others have noticed local improvements at foci not exposed to the rays, which may well be ascribed to general increase in the organic powers of resistance through the action of the rays.

Budde divides the various forms of tuberculosis into superficial and deep-seated. In the former he includes the dermatological forms and lymphomata close to the surface of the body, and in the latter all other forms. Differences in the reaction to the rays are merely a question of degree. According to Budde's observations, the lymphatic glands have far greater power of reaction to the treatment than cases of tuberculosis of the bones even in its surface forms (*e.g.*, *spina ventosa*), probably owing to the special light affinity of the lymphatic tissues as in X-ray treatment.

The best measure of success in the treatment of superficial tuberculosis is provided by lymphomata of the neck and shoulder regions. Budde distinguishes three clinical forms of these, viz.,

(1) the simple hyperplastic form ;

(2) the closed form accompanied by caseation and softening ; and

(3) ulcerated lymphomata with sinuses.

Very similar to the first-named form are the glandular swellings observed after certain infectious diseases, such as influenza (Schmieden), after diseases of the jaws or teeth, etc. Satisfactory results by means of artificial Alpine Sun treatment were obtained by Kautz in 52 cases of non-tubercular inflammatory affections of the glands.

In cases under the first group, Budde not infrequently noticed inflammatory symptoms, which, however, soon subsided ; in a few instances, radiation treatment had to be interrupted on account of fever, considerable swelling and great pain after each radiation. After longer treatment the various single glands either disappeared, although sometimes small resistant nodules persisted, or progressive softening set in. The number of refractory cases belonging to this group is fairly considerable, amounting as it does to about 30%. A combination with deep X-ray treatment is advisable. It would appear that there is a certain antagonism between the two methods, inasmuch as the lymphomata which remain unaffected by ultra-violet rays are rapidly absorbed or softened if treated by X-rays.

It is, in Budde's opinion, a successful result of artificial Alpine Sun treatment if such glands soften and form cold abscesses, thereby passing to the second group mentioned above. The resorption which is the desideratum ensues if the radiations are continued for a sufficiently long time, and can be accelerated by puncture, iodoform-glycerine injections, or by incisions. A decrease in the tendency to form " packets " of glands, *i.e.*, the isolation of the individual glands from the large inflammatory tumorous mass, is always a favourable sign. The effect of artificial Alpine Sun treatment on cases belonging to this group, it is gratifying to note, is consistently good.

Generally speaking, the same holds good for the third group. Deep-seated accumulations of glands with long sinuses are very refractory, requiring powerful protracted radiation, and often combination with X-ray treatment and surgical operations. In the case of superficial infiltrations the effect is nearly always satisfactory. It is least so if there are foci of long standing, embedded in hard fibrous tissue, but most successful in the case of very level forms resembling tuberculous skin ulcers. In addition to general, local radiations have also been used. Treatment should last from five minutes to half-an-hour, at a distance of 20 to 8 inches, covering up other parts if necessary.

The dermatological forms of tuberculosis, ranging from scrofulous eczema to secondary scrofuloderm and the pronounced types of lupus with sinuses, are very suitable subjects for artificial Alpine Sun treatment. X-ray treatment, and above all any measures affecting the deep-seated foci, especially in cases of lupus with sinuses embedded in callous tissue, are of valuable assistance. Certain cures by artificial Alpine Sun treatment may be expected in mild cases. General radiations are the rule, powerful stimulation or other therapeutic measures being required only in exceptional cases.

The speed of healing in cases of superficial tuberculosis is subject to considerable individual variations. On an average six weeks will pass before any distinct effect is apparent. Final healing requires correspondingly longer time if the normal course is followed ; it may be hastened by suitable measures, such as those indicated above.

The benign, serous form of simple *peritonitis tuberculosa*, not complicated by organic disease, tends to disappear even if only the ordinary tonic measures are applied. The artificial Alpine Sun treatment materially aids these measures, as has been confirmed by Strahlmann, Laqueur, Lasser, Ritscher, Selma Mayer, and others. General irradiation is invariably indicated. If tuberculosis of other organs (ileocæcal tuberculosis) is also present, the prognosis is serious ; and the effect of artificial Alpine Sun treatment is correspondingly slight in such cases.

Tuberculous disease of the tendon sheaths, bursæ, bones, and joints, frequently reacts to artificial Alpine Sun treatment at the outset by increasing the swelling, tension and pain, which may be regarded as a reaction of the focus. When these symptoms disappear the patient feels better ; in the forms with sinuses there is a temporary increase of secretion.

The formation of cold abscesses appears to be encouraged by artificial Alpine Sun treatment. König observed this result in cases of vertebral tuberculosis, and Budde in caries of the ribs.

Artificial Alpine Sun radiation is also advantageous in the post-operative treatment of tuberculous cases, *e.g.*, in cases of suppurating sinuses subsequent to resection of the knee joint (König), after extirpation of the sinuses in tuberculosis of the tendon sheaths and the ribs, and more particularly in a serious case of purulent sacro-iliac disease (Budde).

On the whole the local effect of the artificial Alpine Sun treatment upon the tubercular focus is but slight in all these forms, and subject to considerable individual variations. Frischbier obtained the following results in treating various forms of tuberculosis, using both local and general radiation :—

Very good	4·22%
Good	49·15%
Moderate	27·96%
None whatever	18·64%

With the exception of the dermal forms, which are directly accessible to the ultra-violet rays, and affections of the superficial glands, which possess a more than ordinary reactive capacity, the action of the quartz light must be described as indirect. Curative action can only be achieved by the protracted and powerful general radiations. In the majority of cases local improvement does not occur until improvement has occurred in appetite, weight, and mental outlook. Even if no local changes take place, the effects enumerated constitute a considerable success for the treatment, since their presence prepares the ground for applying other therapeutic measures.

In the case of most patients a local action also occurs, shown in the formation of new connective tissue and encystment. The biological energy of the artificial Alpine Sun treatment, however, is not sufficient to cope with cases of destructive tuberculosis of joints, the malignant character of which defies even any other therapeutic measure. According to Strauss, even a tendency of superficial foci to heal may be unfavourably affected by concomitant pulmonary tuberculosis.

The artificial Alpine Sun treatment cannot entirely replace natural heliotherapy, since it lacks the long-waved rays, and the still more important climatic factors Moreover, the long period of time required for a cure involves certain social drawbacks and causes some patients to abandon treatment too soon.

On the other hand, the artificial Alpine Sun treatment possesses certain undeniable advantages. It makes the practitioner, especially in large cities, independent of conditions of weather and cloud. In Budde's opinion, especially with regard to the deep-seated forms of tuberculosis, it is an adjuvant to the conservative and constitutional treatment of the disease, rather than a specific remedy. In combination with the open-air and sunlight treatment, X-ray, therapy venous stasis, orthopædic surgery, tuberculin, etc., its effects are distinctly good.

Schönbauer,* availing himself of the vast material at the Von Eiselsberg Clinic, had special opportunities of studying the effects of quartz light treatment upon tuberculosis of the joints, bones, and glands, diseases which have spread enormously since the war. These effects are particularly good as regards superficial forms, particularly tuberculosis of the glands. If no results could be obtained after several artificial Alpine Sun radiations, the Kromayer Lamp is used as well. The results obtained in tuberculosis of the bones and joints were not quite so favourable as those in glandular tuberculosis, but even here the percentage of cures amounted to 42-44%. The quartz lamp radiation of tuberculous glands is preferable to X-ray treatment, inasmuch as it is absolutely free from any danger, and may be used by any physician without difficulty.

Lexer† regards heliotherapy as the principal remedy in the conservative treatment of surgical tuberculosis, replacing it by artificial Alpine Sun treatment during the winter months.

Riedel,‡ whose paper is of outstanding value, concludes that

*Mitteilungen aus dem Grenzgebiet der Medizin und Chirurgie, vol. xxxiii. No. 4, 1921.

†Deutsche Medizinische Wochenschrift, No. 29, 1921.

‡Strahlentherapie, vol. xii., No. 2.

satisfactory curative results—although not so good as those obtained in the Alps—can be obtained in treating of surgical tuberculosis in high altitudes by using heliotherapy, combined with quartz light radiation on sunless days, and powerful ultra-violet treatment during the winter months. He lays down that the radiation treatment should always be used in conjunction with other methods hitherto approved.

Hagedorn* holds that the effect of artificial Alpine Sun treatment in cases of surgical tuberculosis is merely a general one, tending to improve the patient's condition. With the exception of a few cases of glandular tuberculosis, he has not noticed any specific results, but he considers irradiation altogether superior to X-ray treatment, when treating infantile cases of closed surgical tuberculosis. If ordinary precautions be taken, proper selection made, and due regard paid to the sensitiveness of the skin to ultra-violet rays, even very young children may be exposed for hours together during weeks, and even months, to the vivifying ultra-violet rays.

Staphylococci, radiated with ultra-violet light, are more readily absorbed by the leucocytes and more rapidly destroyed, than non-radiated. Phagocytosis is also stimulated by the simultaneous radiation of the blood and the bacteria.†

Riedel‡ reports good results in the treatment of surgical tuberculosis by combined general radiations with the artificial Alpine Sun and the Sollux lamp. He prefers this combination to the sole use of the former.

Conservative irradiation treatment of light cases of surgical tuberculosis and lupus can also be carried out during consulting hours if admission to a sanatorium or hospital is impossible. Rauschning reports on thirty cases which he successfully treated in this way. He obtained best results with the Sollux lamp as a source of luminous heat (hyperæmia therapy). In addition, the artificial Alpine Sun was important as a general tonic and also as the means, partly specific in its action, to a permanent cure.

Combined Therapy and its Possibilities.

Investigations of the problem of increasing the reactive capacity of the human organism seem to open up future possibilities for

*Würzburger Abhandlungen, vol. xx., Nos. 7 to 9, 1920.
†Azzi Haematologica, vol. i., p. 435.
‡Strahlentherapie, vol. xiii., 1922.

irradiation therapy. These investigations are based on Neuberg's theory of the photosensitive systems (*cf.* the chapter on the sensibility of the skin to ultra-violet rays in individuals), and on Von Tappeiner's hypothesis of the photo-dynamic phenomena. The combination of artificial Alpine Sun and Lekutyl treatment, as recommended by Strauss, may be similarly regarded. Hufnagel has endeavoured to obtain by internal doses of resorcin the conversion of the rays which Rollier ascribes to the presence of pigment. Accepting Neuberg's views, he also prescribes iron, and in the case of patients suffering from advanced anæmia, arsenic as well. He mentions the striking fact that not one of the patients subjected to this treatment showed any signs of a skin reaction subsequent to the radiations, a fact which he ascribes to the effect of the resorcin.

Spiess and Feldt have reported successful results in treating tuberculosis by the use of Jesionek's auro-cantharidin simultaneously with the artificial Alpine Sun treatment. They ascribe the increased physical power and more rapid pigmentation, in cases which prove refractory when treated exclusively by the radiation method, to the components of "Auro-canthan," both of which are activants of oxygenation, the drug being reduced in the organism to colloidal gold.

Dreyer's method of skin sensitization by means of intra- and subcutaneous injections of $1^o/_{oo}$ erythrosin solution, gave for the most part negative therapeutic results (*cf.* Neisser, Halberstädter, Forchhammer, Spiethoff). Better results were obtained by the application of a 5% eosin solution upon ulcers in places where the diseased tissue could absorb the solution (Jesionek).

The use of enzytol, which possesses the property of chemically imitating certain of the effects of radiation, may possibly increase the effect of light, as of X-rays (*cf.* Baisch and others). It is, however, essential to take into account the enhanced sensitiveness of the skin consequent upon the use of such sensitizers, and to exercise special precaution in the radiation treatment.

In order to increase the effect of the light, several authorities have combined artificial Alpine Sun treatment with diathermic therapy.

Hufnagel, Mendel and others obtained good results on the patient's general condition, and on the healing of wounds, by using the Schittenhelm " Condensor Couch " ; and Becker made successful use of this combination when treating serious X-ray injuries.

The combination of artificial Alpine Sun and X-ray treatment has recently become prominent. The action of the former, predominantly of a general character, supplements the local effects of deep X-ray therapy. Possibly each group of rays sensitizes the tissues for the other. Budde warmly recommends this combination.

According to this writer, light filters are unnecessary in general radiation, but for local treatment may be used to diminish the intensity of quartz light applied in surgery. In order to maintain the stimulating effect of the artificial Alpine Sun light on cellular activity, and to eliminate its necrotic effect, Jesionek, Heusner, and others recommend the use of small doses of filtered quartz light to promote the growth of epithelium.

Hufnagel and others obtained good results from the use of light baths. In order to produce a light bath resembling natural sunlight, it is necessary to employ other lamps besides the artificial Alpine Sun, such as the Sollux lamp, or Hagemann's ring of bulbs. These have one property in common with all other sources of light which emit long wave rays in great intensity (*e.g.*, the carbon arc lamp) in the deep penetration of the heat rays they produce. For many purposes it is most advantageous to be thus enabled to evoke a deep hyperæmia without restriction of dosage through the limited toleration of the skin to short wave rays. Such considerations have led Laqueur, Breiger, and others to use the carbon arc light, with or without red or blue filters, for local radiation of wounds in combination with general radiations with the artificial Alpine Sun.

NATURAL AND ARTIFICIAL SUNLIGHT AND CLIMATIC TREATMENT
OF TUBERCULOSIS.

The question which kind of rays are accountable for the successes of treating tuberculosis by light, and what effects are due to other climatic factors, may according to modern views be answered as follows :—

Without doubt, natural sunlight treatment, owing to the other climatic factors mentioned in the introduction, to which may also be added the purity of the air in the mountains and at the sea, has great advantages over treatment with artificial sources of light. But it would be difficult to decide whether there is any climate which is particularly potent in curing tuberculosis ; on the one hand, all resorts for tuberculous patients, with the most various climates, report successes ; on the other, tuberculosis attacks the natives in any climate, even in the high mountains, at the seaside, and in the south, which are specially recommended for tuberculous subjects. Among the natives of southern climates, indeed, tuberculosis is usually more severe in its incidence and leads more rapidly to a fatal issue than in temperate climates.

From this, it can scarcely be assumed that any one climate has specific healing properties against tuberculosis, but rather that the stimulating effects and curative results of climatic cures are probably due to the change, and disappear as soon as the patient has become accustomed to the new climate.

The beneficial influence of the change of climate was very marked in the case of a consumptive patient who, after spending some winters at Davos, went to Chile, whence he paid a visit to Germany every now and then. He had contracted the disease at the age of 20, and had repeatedly had serious hæmorrhage, and relapses during several years. The frequent change between the Alpine climate, mild and sunny climate of Chile, and the bracing effects of sea voyages, however, so favourably affected the disease that he was gradually completely cured and, despite arduous professional work, is still quite fit at the age of 60.

The contrast between Alpine climate and that of the sea appears particularly effective if the change over is brought about gradually and with precaution. Climatic effect is not restricted to respiration but extends also to the functions of the skin ; which, as shown by atonic condition and tendency to perspiration, are mostly deficient in consumptive patients.

Moreover, the change of scenery and surroundings connoted by change of climate is a psychological factor of no small importance. Most tuberculous patients, owing to the compulsory rest and inactivity, are neurasthenic, and suffer from the monotony inseparable from a protracted stay in one locality. Thus, a change of scenery is bound to act as a mental stimulant, provided always that the patient's powers of physical endurance allow it.

Natural insolation treatment forms part of the climatic " cure." In this case, too, allowance must be made for what the patient is accustomed to. Generally speaking, those who are little used to sunshine respond to insolation more freely than those who have grown up in a sunny climate. The experiences gained with artificial Alpine Sun treatment are very similar. Its action, favourable at first, declines if quartz light radiations are applied for months without a break. This is due to the fact that the short-waved ultra-violet rays are obstructed by the increased pigmentation caused by radiation, so that part of their action is lost. Since, in the case of both natural and artificial light baths, ultra-violet light is the chief curative factor, it is advisable not to continue the radiations uninterruptedly for months, but rather to break off after one or two months' treatment, and to resume after an interval of three to four weeks, so that the skin, and also the entire system, may regain reactivity to the ultra-violet rays.

In applying both natural and artificial light treatment to tuberculous patients distinction must be made on the one hand between the treatment of internal and of external or surgical tuberculosis ; and between general radiations, i.e., the sunlight bath, and local radiations on the other.

Local radiations are used in the treatment of surgical tuberculosis. Whenever it is desired to bring about a powerful stimulation of tuberculous ulcers with soft granulations, the best results are obtained by the use of irritative ultra-violet rays below 3000 A.U., which the artificial Alpine Sun lamp emits in greater amount than natural mountain sunshine itself (Jüngling). If, however, it is intended to produce a local hyperæmia, it is preferable to make use of the deep-penetrating ultra-violet rays above 3000 A.U.* in conjunction with the red heat rays; which means either natural sunlight treatment, or a combination of the artificial Alpine Sun with the Sollux lamp or Hagemann lamp ring with the Uviol filter to keep off the irritative rays. Kisch† recommends the use of compression treatment in conjunction with such radiations and with administration of iodine in the form of sodium iodide.

General radiations, i.e., natural and artificial light baths, in addition to local treatment, are beneficial in every form of tuberculosis, including external. Practical experience tends to show

---

* Jünglin g.

† *Münchener Medizinische Wochenschrift*, No. 45, 1919 : Zur Frage der Behandlung der äusseren Tuberkulose ("On the Treatment of Surgical Tuberculosis ").

that the principal effect of general radiations upon tuberculosis is due to the action of the ultra-violet rays. No matter whether we give preference to the irritative ultra-violet rays, to the penetrative rays of the artificial Alpine Sun, or to natural insolation, the result will always be dependent upon the amount of ultra-violet present. It follows that the results obtainable from treatment with natural sunlight in low altitudes—which contains ultra-violet only in small amount—can never be as good as those obtainable by the natural or artificial Alpine sun, because the main difference between the natural and artificial Alpine sun on the one hand, and lowland sunlight on the other, does not consist in the other climatic factors, but exclusively in the percentage of ultra-violet rays present. The undeniable results achieved by Rollier and Bernhard are solely attributable to the greater amount of ultra-violet rays present in Alpine sunlight, as has been proved by the investigations of Dorno.* Hence it is not sufficient merely to warn against undue expectations from natural insolation treatment, as Brüning does, but rather the fact should be emphasized that any source of light which is deficient in ultra-violet can only produce very limited results.

To what extent red light assists the action of ultra-violet, is another question, to answer which connotes some consideration of individual skin reactive capacity to light. I have repeatedly emphasized the importance of this point, and given expression to my belief that the influence of the radiations upon the organism as a whole consists in their effect on the excretive function of the skin and its regulation of bodily heat, or in other words in the improvement of the self-adjusting functions of the skin.†

If we agree with Hoffman's theory‡ that "the skin possesses a special biological function—esophylaxis—by means of which it can produce protective and curative substances assisting the internal organs and nervous system against the attacks of noxious germs and their poison, and protect them from these enemies to the system," my own views are not only corroborated, but we are

*c.f. Physik der Sonnen- und Himmelstrahlung (" The Physical Aspects of Sunlight "), contributed to *Strahlentherapie*, vols. ix. and x., 1919.

†cf Beitrag zur Wirkung der künstlichen Höhensonne auf die Haut und ihre Funktionen, published in No. 22 of the *Münchener Medizinische Wochenschrift*, 1919.

‡cf. Über eine nach innen gerichtete Schutzfunktion der Haut : Esophylaxie (" Esophylaxis : A Function of the Skin Affecting the Internal Organs "), published in No. 45 of the *Deutsche Medizinische Wochenschrift*, 1919.

also in a position to account for the part played by the skin in the immunization of the whole organism against the carriers of infection. Since the skin of tuberculous patients is mostly thin, flaccid, and easily inclined to perspiration, and since the effect of ultra-violet is to make it firmer and drier, thus exercising a stimulating influence upon its excretive power and heat regulation, its treatment by red rays without ultra-violet cannot be successful to any degree. Moreover, an essential factor contributing to a successful result is the formation of pigment, and only the ultra-violet rays, but not the red, have this effect. The primary indication for treatment of tuberculous patients is therefore sun baths containing an abundance of ultra-violet light, which means natural or artificial Alpine Sun baths.

This view is apparently contradicted by the results achieved by Reyn*, who reports that the results obtained from treating lupus by means of carbon arc light were better than those obtained with the artificial Alpine Sun. He mentions, however, nothing concerning the condition and the functions of the skin of his patients, and in the absence of such information it cannot be said with certainty whether carbon arc light is in every case preferable to artificial Alpine Sun treatment of lupus, particularly since Jesionek reports good results from treating lupus by means of the latter. But even although, in many cases, the combined application of red and ultra-violet rays may appear better, it still remains that ultra-violet is indispensable in all cases.

In all cases and forms of tuberculosis, we must realize that it is primarily the organism itself which possesses powers by which healing is effected, and that, like all other remedies, natural and artificial light baths as well as climate can only serve more or less to stimulate and assist these natural powers. No remedy, not even a surgical operation, can be relied upon to be effective, if these powers fail. Where they are, however, capable of improvement, successes will be obtained by natural and artificial light baths and climatic cures in the treatment of all forms of tuberculosis superior to those yet achieved by any other method. Patients who are obliged to live in large cities and suffer from bad air, lack of

*Die Resultate der Behandlung mit kunstlichen, chemischen Lichtbaedern bei Lupus vulgaris und chirugischer Tuberkulose (" The Results obtained from the treatment of Lupus Vulgaris and Surgical Tuberculosis by means of Artificial—Chemical—Sources of Light "), published in vol. x., No. 1, of *Strahlentherapie.*

sufficient sunshine, inadequate food and attention, benefit from a sunlight and climatic cure even in the lowlands, although the sunlight of low altitudes contains little ultra-violet. A typical illustration of this is furnished by the successful results which Bier* and his assistant Kisch achieved at Hohenlychen in treating surgical tuberculosis.

These two authors, however, are certainly wrong in denying altogether in their report and elsewhere (*cf.* the publications of Kisch quoted in this book) the efficacy of the violet and ultra-violet rays, and in stating that artificial Alpine Sun treatment is devoid of any curative influence whatever, ascribing their successes solely to the sunlight of the plain (more especially to the red heat rays) and to the climate of Hohenlychen, which according to Bier is one of the best in the world. They omit to take into account the fact that their tuberculous patients came from Berlin, where they were deprived of pure air and sunshine and probably underfed, so that, in their case, the plentiful supply of bright sunshine would in itself be sufficient to exercise an extremely beneficial influence apart from the specific effects of ultra-violet light. The red heat rays of lowland sunlight are certainly useful, as has been said, where hyperæmia is required, but the effect of the ultra-violet of the natural or the artificial Alpine Sun on the organism as a whole cannot be replaced by the red heat rays ; and, indeed, as stated in my paper,† I have pointed out that these played a by no means unimportant part in the illuminants used at Hohenlychen, even though present in slight extent. Moreover, the results obtained at Hohenlychen are in no small measure due to change of surroundings, to abundance of bright sunshine and pure air, and to the good food and proper attendance provided for the patients. Excellent proof that ultra-violet rays are indispensable when treating tuberculosis by light is given by Bier and Kisch themselves, for at the University Surgical Clinic (in the Ziegelstrasse), where they are both active, Alpine Sun quartz lamps have been used since 1912 for treating surgical tuberculosis, with the best results.

*cf. *Tuberkulosis*, vol. xvii., Nos. 10-12, 1918.

†Beitrag zur Wirkung der künstlichen Höhensonne auf die Haut und ihre Funktionen (" On the Effect of Artificial ' Alpine Sun ' Treatment upon the Skin and its Functions "), *Münchener Medizinische Wochenschrift*, No. 22, 1919.

From the foregoing considerations, the following technique is valid for the treatment of tuberculosis by natural and artificial light and climate :—

(1) Occasional change of climate, and periodical break in application of natural or artificial light treatment may be recommended.

(2) A specific effect upon the organism as a whole is solely attributable to the ultra-violet rays.

(3) Only such radiation sources may be expected to bring about successful results as contain an abundance of ultra-violet light. Hence, lowland sunlight is not a substitute for natural or artificial Alpine sun treatment.

(4) Regard must always be paid to the condition and functions of the individual skin.

(5) Lasting success can only be achieved if the natural recuperative powers of the body are still capable of response.

—— ——

Summary.

Artificial Alpine Sun treatment has proved successful in the following surgical conditions :—

In aseptic operation wounds ; and further, in wounds made under non-aseptic conditions, radiation accelerates the process of healing by stimulating vascularization, and also favourably influences the nutrition of small skin flaps with narrow pedicles.

In cicatrization it promotes the formation of fine scars, and has a beneficial and softening effect upon keloids.

In clean, superficial, contused flesh wounds associated with serious damage and destruction to the surrounding tissue, radiation stimulates secretion, promotes hyperæmia, deodorizes the wounds, and facilitates demarcation and the elimination of necrotic tissues. The same holds good for injuries caused by serious primary infections, for paronychia, boils, carbuncles, etc.

With clean, well granulating wounds, mild radiations assist the process of natural healing.

With torpid and soft granulations (*ulcus cruris*, secondary syphilitic ulcers, etc.), powerful radiations are of value.

In wounds complicated by injuries to bones, radiation promotes the elimination of foreign bodies, and accelerates the sequestration of dying bone particles.

With tuberculous and syphilitic wounds general radiations are useful not only for the healing of the wounds and the formation of callus, but also for strengthening the debilitated organism.

In metabolic disturbances caused by vascular cramp and arteriosclerosis (senile gangrene, frost-bite, burns, chemical burns), they hasten the restoration of normal circulation and promote demarcation.

Wounds infected by *bacillus pyocyaneus*, erysipelas, tetanus, and the so-called " latent infection " ; resorption of extravasations and the absorption of fluid accumulations. In these cases, and in the case of specific exudates such as *empyema pleuræ*, they facilitate vascularization.

Peritonitis tuberculosa, especially the serous form and all kinds of surgical tuberculosis (lymphomata, tendon sheaths, membranes, bones and joints, cold abscesses), and for the after-care of these diseases, prolonged powerful general radiations are recommended.

Lymphomata of other kinds and swollen glands after other diseases.

General radiations, applied in addition to local, improve the patients' general condition, and indirectly promote the cure of the local disease.

CHAPTER III.

PEDIATRICS.

By Dr. Ferdinand Rohr.

I. Indications.

The following presents a short summary of what appears, from my knowledge of the literature and from my own experience, worth mentioning regarding the use of the artificial Alpine Sun quartz lamp in the domain of pediatrics.

---

1. Rickets.

In my opinion this disease constitutes a domain for artificial Alpine Sun treatment. Huldschinsky, who first made exact observations on this subject, ascribes a specific effect to irradiation. Whilst the first observations concerning rickets were made in the domain of therapeutics, it was not long before clinical experience and experiments on animals showed that prophylactic irradiation against this disease is also of very pronounced effectiveness.

(a) *Prophylactic Irradiation.*

A number of writers (*e.g.*, Hamburger) are of the opinion that it is possible, by means of proper nourishment, phosphated cod-liver oil, and abundance of fresh air, to conduct prophylactic treatment of rickets which is absolutely adequate in a clinical sense. Others, on the contrary (*e.g.*, Birk and Schall), hold that certain and complete prevention of rickets cannot be achieved by such measures, a view which I am inclined to share.

Putzig was the first to point out the excellent prophylactic effect of artificial Alpine Sun radiation with regard to rickets, having achieved good results on prematurely-born infants. These were confirmed by other investigators ; Mengert, in particular, urges prophylactic irradiation of premature, puny, and syphilitic babies.

Birk and Schall report their successes in large scale treatment. In an institution with 40 infant cases, rickets increased continuously during the winter of 1920-21, despite unbroken administration of phosphated cod-liver oil. The increase was checked from Dec. 1st, when, in addition to the oil, irradiation and fresh vegetable juices were given ; inside three and a half weeks, rickets was unknown in the Institution. An epidemic of whooping cough having caused discontinuance of irradiation (for technical reasons), the rickets reappeared. Next winter, in addition to the oil and vegetable juices, irradiation was administered with the arc lamp (Spektrosol lamp), but no prophylactic action on rickets could be established.

Powers, Park, Shipley, McCollum, and Simmonds confirm the preventive action of quartz light in rickets by experiments on rats fed on a rickets-producing diet. The radiated animals remained free of rickets, while the controls developed the disease severely in all cases.

Hess and his collaborators, as well as Schultzer and Sonne, also write on similar lines.

Powerful irradiation protects black and white animals equally, but weaker irradiation only the white and not the black, the latter showing lower blood calcium content. The investigators explain the greater susceptibility of the American negro to rickets hereby. Kramer and his colleagues were unable to confirm this distinction, though not in a prophylactic, yet in a therapeutic sense, between white men and black.

The further experiments of Hess deserve mention, which established that irradiation did not prevent rickets in rats when the rays had been filtered through window glass 4 mm. thick, but with a thickness of 2 mm. speedy prevention of rickets occurred. Filtration of rays through woollen or cotton fabrics allowed a range of results from good to poor, according to the wideness of the mesh.

Schultzer and Sonne established that radiation did not prevent rickets in rats when ultra-violet rays were filtered out through a container filled with quinine bi-sulphate ; this may, perhaps, be explained by the action of glass alone as described above. When filtered through Uviol glass, which absorbs only the shorter ultra-violet, the protective action remained ; the rays of wave-length between 4000 and 2800 A.U. are therefore the active components of the spectrum. For the rest, the effects were the same whether the animals were radiated for a quarter of an hour or only two to five minutes daily.

Pappenheimer's view deserves mention, which conceives

McCollum's experimental " Ca-deficient rickets " not as this disease proper, but as an osteoporosis ; for the rest, however, this writer holds both forms of rickets as most favourably responsive to quartz light, both in the prophylactic and therapeutic sense.

It may now be taken as proven, that a reasonably certain prophylaxis of rickets was only achieved with the introduction of the artificial Alpine Sun among the preventive measures. It is advisable for all children liable to rickets from bad housing or other family conditions, and particularly for premature babies and twins, no matter whether breast or bottle-fed ; and this is more especially the case during the winter and spring. If irradiation be combined with the customary therapeutic measures, prevention of rickets is so probable as to border on certainty (Birk and Schall). Irradiation is given for a period suited to the needs of the case (*see* under " Technique ").

(b) Therapeutic Irradiation.

Huldschinsky checked the effects of artificial Alpine Sun irradiation on bone formation by skiagrams, and his conclusion is that quartz light therapy is absolutely successful in treating rickets, and effective at all stages without exception.

Great importance is ascribed to the blood-chemistry of rickets, which can also be used to check results achieved in treatment.

In the florid stage a marked deficiency of inorganic serum phosphorus is always present ; the more pronounced the disease, the greater the diminution of phosphorus-content of the serum ; while as healing progresses this content is restored to normal. The rapidity of metabolic restoration, measured in this respect, is the same under quartz light radiation as under phosphorated cod-liver oil treatment (Kramer, Casparis, Howland) ; a normal phosphorus content is often reached in three to four weeks, but as a rule requires two months. There is usually strict parallelism between the inorganic phosphorus serum content and the other rachitic symptoms.

The observations of Scheer and Salomon, György, Hess, Gutmann, Jundell, are similar.

Controverting the observations of earlier writers who found increased calcium-content accompanying rickets, recent investigators (Howland and Kramer, György, Kneschke, Tisdall) have not confirmed this, but found rather normal values often with a tendency to decrease. When improvement sets in, the serum calcium content, which is often lowered, increases slowly to the normal count of 10 to 11 mg. per cent. ; according to R. Mayer, the blood-calcium decreases somewhat during the first days of irradiation, subsequently increasing.

The low retention of calcium and phosphorus characteristic of rickets is, according to Lasch, increased by ultra-violet irradiation. This increase sets in strikingly soon after the commencement of treatment and persists some time after clinical cure of the disease has taken place. The rapidity with which improvement commences leads him to conclude that the morbid process in rickets cannot consist in retrogressive pathological changes, but that disturbances of the intermediary metabolic changes are concerned. This striking improvement in the deficient lime and phosphorus retention in rickets is confirmed by American writers (Orr, Holt, Wilkins, Boone).

Attention has been drawn to the effect of artificial Alpine Sun irradiation on another metabolic disturbance characteristic of rickets, the increased intermediate acid-formation and consequent acid-excretion, signs of metabolic retardation. The action of irradiation is to decrease this.

Whilst clinical experience has at all times ascribed great importance to natural sunlight treatment, the first " chemical " evidence of a reversal of the metabolism thereby has only recently been given by Hess and Gutmann, who, by means of sun-bathing rickety infants for half-an-hour to an hour daily, raised the blood phosphate values from their sub-normal level of between 2·77 and 3·7 mg. per cent. to normal (4·05 to 4·8 mg. per 100 grams of blood) in a period of two to four months. This result, which only confirms clinical experience, merits close comparison with mercury quartz light treatment in regard to length and frequency of the individual radiations, and the duration of healing. It would almost appear as if natural sunlight, of which quartz light is frequently regarded as a mere substitute, had no great advantages over the latter, which would yield at least equal results in an equal period with shorter and less frequent radiations, can be more accurately administered for dosage, and moreover is available at all times. Lestocquoy also holds that ultra-violet therapy is more rapidly effective than sunlight treatment, as does S. Rosenbaum, who concludes, from check experiments made in the Leipzig

Children's Clinic, that "natural sunlight, having regard to our climatic limitations, manifests pronounced curative power, which, however, does not come up to that of the artificial Alpine Sun."

Huldschinsky's observations have shown that the time required for complete cure varies with the stage of the disease present. Each stage requires its own course of treatment and time for cure. From this point of view he distinguishes five stages, viz. :—

(1) Incipient decalcification—during the child's first year of life—cured in one or two months.

(2) Incipient passive osteoid formations, *i.e.*, the mild form of florid rickets—during the first and second years— cured in two or three months.

(3) Maximum degree of passive osteoid formations, *i.e.*, the acute form of florid rickets—second and third years— cured in from three to six months.

(4) Torpid or stationary stage, the processes of formation and destruction more or less balanced, *i.e.*, the mild form of inveterate rickets—third and fourth years— cured in from four to seven months.

(5) Active osteoid formations, *i.e.*, the acute form of inveterate rachitic osteomalacia—after the fourth year— cured in from six to nine months.

Roughly speaking, the cure takes as many months as the number of years the child is old (Huldschinsky and L. F. Meyer). The healing process can be followed by X-ray photographs simultaneously with the clinical cure. The process is more rapid than by the use of cod-liver oil (according to Huldschinsky and György).

Jundell in particular reports on a comparison of 12 cases, 6 cured by irradiation and 6 by dietetic treatment, the duration of cure being the same for all ; this report should, however, be weighted in favour of irradiation treatment, owing to the fact that the cases were so treated during the winter months, the others during the period April to July—spontaneous cure !

Pflüger speaks of results with the artificial Alpine Sun after a course lasting two to three weeks as equal to those after two to three months of phosphorated cod-liver oil. The effect is retroactive. Craniotabes is quickly healed ; advanced degrees of softening of widest extension ossify firmly within three weeks.

Craniotabes is the most simple clinical test of successful results, since they can be measured from time to time by means of a diagram or measurements of the area of softening. It must, however, be noted that a definite cure as established by skiagrams or by measurement of the serum-phosphate content requires longer than clinical cure of the craniotabes ; on this account Birk and Schall recommend that irradiation should be prolonged even after clinical cure has occurred. R. Hamburger, who holds that the cause of rickets lies in the sum of several lime-reducing factors, terms the action of irradiation " lime-stabilizing." In addition to the ossification, irradiation also affects the *spasmus nutans*, perspiration, pain and tendency to pneumonia. On the other hand, no perceptible decrease in the size of the fontanelles can be proved. Teething and growth are promoted. Anæmia, despite healing of the bones, is not greatly improved.

The fact that children in whom the bones, as shown by Röntgenograms, are completely cured, are sometimes a long time before they begin to walk is explained by Huldschinsky on the grounds that the ability to walk has been lost through the long illness and not as due to a continuance of the illness. After some time the children invariably learn to walk in due course, and this can also be accelerated by exercises to strengthen the muscles of locomotion.

Karger extends the meaning of the term cerebral rickets coined by Czerny and Keller, which comprises all the nervous symptoms of the disease, and uses it in contradistinction to that of osseous rickets. His assertion that, according to his observations, the ultra-violet rays are effective only on the latter, is sharply disputed by Huldschinsky on the basis of his own experience in 105 cases.

Until recently treatment of rickets consisted in allowing the disease to heal and then operating on the deformed bones when hardened. Huldschinsky, on the other hand, recommended a bloodless operation on the soft bone in conjunction with simultaneous radiations, since it is quite possible to allow the bone to harden after it has been straightened and whilst still in plaster. Wehner and Jacobsen recommended " taking rickety leg deformities of advanced degree in the florid or healing stage, correcting and remodelling, if necessary after preliminary softening of the bones in plaster-of-Paris, and irradiation with ultra-violet light after correction has taken place." Riedel, of the Ludloff Clinic, confirms the beneficial effect of quartz light upon the rachitic bone process, but rejects surgical measures, if X-rays show that the florid stage is still present. He argues that in cases where these have been carried out, less satisfactory results were achieved, and the healing was considerably delayed.

According to Huldschinsky, the healing process continues spontaneously after one month's radiation in the first and second stages, and after two months in the third stage, whereas in the serious cases of the fourth and fifth stages, the healing tendency diminishes, and necessitates renewed radiations.

On the evidence of 200 cases, he proved that success was invariable, and quicker than by the former methods. He recommended a course of two months' treatment for children under two years old, and for those over that age, three months' treatment, four weeks' break, and renewed radiation in the fifth month. These successes were confirmed by all writers (Birk and Schall, Michaelis, L. F. Meyer, Erlacher, Hamburger, Gracia Donato, Rosenstern, Jundell, Riedel, Rohr, Weber, Marchionini, and others). Weltring describes the experiences of the Würzburg Kinderklinik, where four to six weeks' intensive radiation, succeeded by cod-liver oil treatment till the spring, sufficed to heal rickets and to guard against relapses.

As concerns attempts to explain these facts, it has been shown that damage arising from alimentary disorders can be influenced by the action of light ; this follows indubitably from the observations of German and American authors, partly summarized above. Opinions differ on the question of how this established effect of light on metabolism takes place. Birk and Schall conceive its action as analagous to that of vitamins on the bones, favouring the assimilation of calcium. Freudenberg and György concur ; they assume that in rickets a disturbance of the osseous calcium–ion fixation takes place, evoked through an acidosis. On the basis of the diminished phosphate-serum-content, of the increased phosphate excretion, the markedly high amount of ammonia in the urine and the diminished alkali reserve characteristic of rickets, they arrive at the conception that acidosis is the expression of a retardation of metabolism. Acidosis-causing foods (butter fat, for example) intensify this, whereas metabolic stimulants such as irradiation and vitamines lead to cure.

Others regard the action of light as a kind of " protoplasm

activation." The reduction products arising from irradiation affect the bones in the direction of improved bone assimilation. It was established by Eckstein and von Möllendorf that dyes introduced into the skin of animals were dispersed quicker in irradiated than non-radiated subjects ; in their view owing to more intense flushing of the skin by blood, through irradiation. Their conception of " protoplasm activation " through the decomposition products caused by irritation of the skin cannot be fully reconciled with the observations of Sachs, who failed to produce any effect on rickets by the therapy of irritative protein-bodies (caseosan ; horse-serum).

Rothmann and Callenberg, investigating the action of artificial Alpine Sun quartz light on the serum calcium condition, believe that the action of irradiation consists in a paralyzing of the sympathetic system of the skin, causing movement of calcium away from the skin, which shows itself in increase of the serum-calcium content.

Contradicting these views, which are based on the theory of radiation effect on the outermost layers of the skin, Levy and Gassul speak rather of deep-seated action, from their experiments, which, however, are not held as authoritative from the pediatric standpoint.

Pigmentation appears to play no part at least in rickets (cf. the observations of Kramer and Hess on human and animal subjects).

More recent investigations show that the same anti-rachitic effects are produced in animals and men by the administration of irradiated cholesterin containing foodstuffs (milk, flour, etc., skin) as by direct radiation. These point to the assumption that in the healing of rickets, both by direct irradiation of the body and by means of irradiated food, activated cholesterin (or else a new substance, akin to cholesterin, and produced therefrom by ultra-violet radiation) is to be regarded as the common effective agent in both cases. (See also page 55.)

In experiments on animals, skin irradiated in vitro when given as food was definitely proved to have anti-rachitic properties, whilst non-radiated control specimens had not. (A. F. Hess, György, and Popovicin.)

Agreeing with Huldschinsky, we may regard ultra-violet therapy of rickets as superior to treatment with cod-liver oil, massage, and dietetic regulation, in respect of speed, certainty, exactitude of dosage and applicability at any time. The earlier treatment begins, the shorter its duration, and the more certain the protection from rachitic deformities and affections of the respiratory organs.

(c) *Radiation of Foodstuffs.*

(See also pages 52–55.)

Rickets may be influenced not only by means of direct irradiation, but also by the administration of irradiated foodstuffs.

We owe this discovery to A. F. Hess, Steenbock, and their fellow-workers, who came upon it simultaneously and independently in experiments on white rats. Maintaining a rickets-producing diet, they were able to prevent the outbreak of the disease by the addition of foodstuffs, otherwise inert, but irradiated. In this way various oils, a number of vegetable products, vegetables, and also chemically pure cholesterin and phytosterin were activated and acquired anti-rachitic properties, which manifested themselves by activity even twelve months later. Cholesterin, which occurs in milk, flour, and also in animal and human skin, seems to play a special part in the activation of foodstuffs ; after several hours' radiation its physical properties are distinctly changed (melting point lowered, absorption spectrum altered). Beumer showed that it loses a considerable portion (between 3 and 9·5%) of its power of precipitating digitonin after radiation, which might well signify some alteration in its chemical structure also.

Long-continued radiation (17 to 24 hours) not only destroys the acquired anti-rachitic power given to neutral foodstuffs by radiation, but also takes away the activity from substances originally anti-rachitic, such as cod-liver oil and yolk of egg. This is the best evidence of an identity of the rickets-preventing substance (vitamin D), which is present in cod-liver oil and yolk of egg and is produced by radiation in certain foodstuffs.

Working independently of each other, Cowell, Kramer, and György, whose observations were made upon a large number of patients, were able to demonstrate from experiments on babies that milk gains anti-rachitic properties through radiation with the mercury vapour lamp, and that nutrition with radiated milk brings about healing in every case, which can also be checked by means of X-ray photographs and blood chemical tests.

Hottinger writes in the same favourable sense of radiated mothers' milk and cows' milk.

György radiates the entire day's ration prepared by addition of diluting fluids and of the necessary solids, and ready cooked, for a period of 30 to 60 minutes at a distance of 30 to 40 cms., stirring it frequently during exposure in dishes or bowls. This " jecorized " milk has an " indefinable, slightly musty taste and smell, somewhat resembling cod-liver oil," but children take it and digest it well.

The radiation of ready-prepared milk-food is accompanied by two disadvantages :—

1. It must be radiated daily.

2. The ration must be consumed within twenty-four hours.

On this account the method proposed by György, of using radiated milk powder, constitutes a great advantage. We know from numerous publications that the use of milk powder instead of fresh milk, even when continued over long periods, is unaccompanied by any detriment to the health of infants. (Czerny, Finkelstein, Neuland, Peiper, Nobel, Wagner, György ; American and English writers.)

Radiated milk powder may therefore be used and prescribed freely, and can " accomplish a cure both of florid rickets without complications, and also of tetany in precisely the same time as jecorized fresh milk ; a complete cure as checked by skiagrams and blood-chemistry (with deposits of lime which are visible on X-ray photographs) " (György, 40 cases). These communications of György are confirmed by the simultaneous publications of A. F. Hess (3 cases) and Mackay (2 cases).

The radiated milk powder retains the " induced radiant energy " for a long time (at least four months) unweakened.

György radiates the milk powder, spread out in a thin layer (1–2 mm.), for 45 to 60 minutes, at a distance of 30 cms. After treatment, it is returned to its original tins. Like radiated fresh milk, the treated milk powder has a peculiar rancid taste and odour, but is likewise well taken and digested. György recommends as a precaution at the commencement of a course of treatment, that jecorized milk should not at once be given for all meals, but begun gradually with one bottle a day and increased by one at a time.

Since milk powder prepared according to the Krause process contains little or no vitamins, the amount of anti-scorbutic substance in particular being very small, it is advisable in practice regularly to add vitamins (especially Factor C).

Since Cholesterin, which is so important in the activation of foodstuffs, is primarily bound up with milk fat, the therapeutic or prophylactic use of buttermilk can be of little use, whereas the administration of radiated milk fat seems to promise success. Experiments in this direction have been begun by Ottokarl Schultz and myself, first on rats and next on human subjects, the results of which will be published later ; these have established the remarkable fact that no change of taste occurs when milk fat (cream + butter) is radiated, provided that the constituents have been sufficiently deprived of albumen.* From this we believe ourselves justified in concluding that the impairment of taste through radiation, which György and others regard as a sign of activation of the foods (jecorization), has nothing to do with the process of activation, but is rather due to the decomposition of albuminous substances. This assumption is also supported by the fact that olive oil, which has an albumen content, is changed in taste through radiation, whereas pure triolein does not undergo any such change (*see* also page 52).

2. TETANY.

(Laryngismus Stridulus, Fits, Carpopedal Spasms, and Broncho-Tetany.)

Tetany is another disorder which is eminently suitable for treatment by the mercury quartz lamp, whether latent or already manifest in eclamptic spasms, laryngismus stridulus, carpopedal spasms, or broncho-tetanic symptoms. Mercury vapour light evidently possesses specific action in spasmophilia similar to that possessed by phosphorated cod-liver oil ; whether in greater or lesser degree cannot be stated at present.

In treating infantile tetany, distinction must be made between symptomatic measures with immediate effects—calcium therapy in particular—and those giving permanent results (Freudenberg, György), among which are cod-liver oil and quartz light. For choice, both should be combined. Thus, after irradiation, the

---

*Commercial 20% cream is not sufficiently de-albumenised.

symptoms of tetany disappear in a short time, and the manifestations which often persist after these have gone, the electrical
supersensitivity (Erb's sign) and the facial phenomenon (Chvostek's
sign), return fairly quickly to normal. The period of treatment
necessarily varies from four days to four weeks (Huldschinsky,
Sachs).

Investigation of metabolism in tetany, although there exists an
intimate clinical connection between the disposition to tetany and
the basis of rickets, gives, according to Freudenberg and György,
a reversed image of that in rickets. The serum calcium value,
normal or slightly subnormal in rickets, is greatly lowered, whilst
the serum phosphorus is relatively increased ; the excretion of
acid in the urine, increased in rickets, is lowered ; while the rate
of metabolism, lowered in rickets, is increased ; and so forth.
As artificial Alpine Sun quartz light strongly influences metabolism
in an alkaline sense, over-strong dosage can even increase the
tetanic condition at the outset. Thus Huldschinsky reports of
tetany becoming manifest after powerful irradiation.

The good results from artificial Alpine Sun treatment in cases
of tetany are, in the view of both authors above named, in the
main ascribable to the cure of the basal rickety condition thereby
effected. In a case of laryngospasm under my observation, in
which spasms of the glottis ceased on the day of the second
radiation (the first had taken place two days previously), I
observed a return of the electrical sensitivity to normal values
(cathode opening contraction greater than 5 m. amp. and cessation
of the reverse anodal contraction) and prompt return of the
positive facial phenomenon (Chvostek's sign) to negative.

In another case of mine, treatment by calcium, phosphorus and
cod-liver oil removed the laryngeal spasms and broncho-tetany,
but could not affect the electrical irritability and " facial
phenomenon " ; these, however, became respectively normal and
negative at the third quartz lamp radiation, and even remained
so when the danger of tetanic symptoms again became acute
owing to an intervening attack of broncho-pneumonia (*see* Fig. 21).

In a further case of manifest tetany, in which a fortnight's
phosphorated cod-liver oil treatment had no effect on the electrical
irritability, a control period of nine days without treatment was
interposed, and the irradiation with the quartz light only taken
up when the possibility of after-action from this medicament,

decisively present in the preceding case, was less likely. Here also the irritability returned to normal after four radiations (Fig. 22).

I could not, however, presume yet to evaluate these and similar observations in the sense of a superiority of quartz light treatment

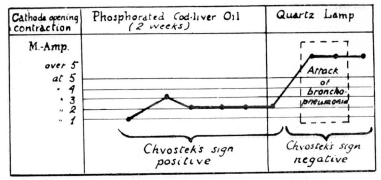

Cathode opening contraction	Phosphorated Cod-liver Oil (2 weeks)	Quartz Lamp
M.-Amp. over 5 at 5 " 4 " 3 " 2 " 1		Attack of broncho-pneumonia
	Chvostek's sign positive	Chvostek's sign negative

FIG. 21.

over the old and approved therapy of phosphorated cod-liver oil. This must be reserved for further investigations.

Benzing, at the Würzburg Children's Clinic, established an increase in the cathodic opening contraction in older children after irradiation, while Weltring, experimenting on many cases

Cathode opening contraction	Phosphorated codliver oil (2 Weeks)	No treatment (9 days)	Quartz Lamp
M Amp over 5 at 5 " 4 " 3 " 2 1			
	Chvostek's sign positive.		Chvostek's sign negative

FIG. 22.

of infantile tetany with remarkably low figures of electrical irritability in many instances, never found an increase of this irritability, testing several times at intervals after each irradiation. Woringer found the blood-calcium values always low in cases of infants with spasmophilia, which returned to normal after three or four weeks of Alpine Sun radiation.

Hoag has communicated some interesting observations, on the basis of which he recommends quartz light as superior to the accepted therapy of calcium and cod-liver oil in both latent and manifest tetany.

He checked the effect by determination of the blood calcium value, taking the return to normal values (10 mg. per cent.) as a sign of cure ; irradiation was administered daily at a distance of 20 inches, beginning with two minutes each on back and front, and increasing by one minute each daily. The dietary consisted of pure or diluted milk, with cereals for older children, but no green vegetables or fruit juices.

In cases of active tetany, steady clinical improvement, which proceeded simultaneously with increased serum calcium values, resulted in a cure in an average time of 41 minutes' irradiation (*i.e.*, in about 13 days) ; in cases of latent tetany, the average was about 60 minutes (*i.e.*, about 16 days). Children used as controls, treated with calcium and cod-liver oil, had not regained normal serum calcium values after six to eight weeks.

Flesch, also, on the basis of successful irradiations in 14 cases, regards quartz light as superior to all other treatments for tetany. Rohmer recommends its use in conjunction with calcium, as in combined lime and cod-liver oil administration.

A more recent German report on the clinical use of quartz light treatment in tetany is by Ruth Stern, of L. F. Meyer's Clinic. Forty-five cases of infantile tetany were given only irradiation with the artificial Alpine Sun in large doses ; 2–3 minutes at 20 inches for the commencement, increasing by 4–6 minutes daily. Cures were effected on the average in 4·8 days' treatment, equalling 50 minutes' actual radiation. Only five relapses occurred : 15 children showed initial set-back, expressed as increased electrical irritability, whilst 2 cases developed severe convulsions or laryngeal spasm, terminating fatally. In consequence of these, whilst recognizing the excellent results, it was suggested that calcium, sal ammoniac, or hydrochloric acid should nightly be added during the first irradiations.

Weltring, of the Würzburg Children's Clinic, reports that " among cases of good effect from irradiation alone others which showed no appreciable improvement after even eight days' intensive irradiation " were observed ; on the other hand Marchionini, at the Leipzig Children's Clinic, had only one failure in 32 cases.

K

From all that has been said it follows that in the quartz mercury vapour lamp we have an important therapeutic adjuvant in fighting infantile tetany, which alone may well lead to success in numerous cases, but whose use should preferably be selected in conjunction with calcium-therapy at the outset (Falkenheim and György), and which, thus used, must be regarded as at least equal, if not superior, to the accepted methods of treatment in tetany.

---

3. INFANTILE TUBERCULOSIS.

A. SURGICAL TUBERCULOSIS.

Schönbauer reports 42–52% of cures by quartz light radiations on a thousand cases of surgical tuberculosis in Vienna during the early post-war years, in spite of extremely unfavourable food conditions.

(a) Lymphadenitis tuberculosa.

The action of the artificial Alpine Sun quartz lamp on the various forms of tubercular glandular swellings is usually very successful, particularly with external glands of the neck positively diagnosed as tuberculous, such as are frequently found in front of the sterno-cleido-mastoid, at the angle of the jaw, and under the chin. If untreated, they generally persist a very long time, sometimes for several years, but by irradiation it is possible in most cases to reduce them considerably. Swellings of the size of a pigeon's egg to a walnut remain either no larger than a cobnut, or as small flat vestiges of fibrous structure. Entire disappearance of the swellings is not usually effected. Infections of the tonsils occasionally causes enlargement of these fibrous lymphomata, which does not always subside when the infection disappears. Whether the coarse fibrous swellings denote a permanent cure is questionable, but the children generally remain healthy for years. The effect of irradiation on glandular concretions is a slow separation of the individual glands from each other until they can finally be felt as isolated knots. Complete return to normal does not as a rule occur. Softening accompanied by an inflammatory erythema is by no means a bad sign. Birk and Schall regard this as particularly advantageous and have finally adopted the technique of working for softening rather than against it.

They anticipate discharge by a small incision at the upper margin of the glands, continuing the irradiation treatment. These successful results in treating tuberculous glands are confirmed by numerous other authors (Michaelis, Weltring, and others). Repeated incision of such soft parts is indicated, and coupled with simultaneous irradiation accelerate healing, leaving only very small—if any—fibrous remnants. Sinuses of softened glands, both spontaneous and artificial, rapidly heal under irradiation, often without adhesions. The usual length of treatment required is two to six months' irradiation (Hamburger). If the sinuses are already of some months' standing at the commencement of the treatment, the results are very much less successful than in fresh cases, and for such it is recommended that combined quartz light and X-ray treatment be adopted, which should be repeated at intervals of three to four weeks. Softened tubercular glands are not as a rule influenced towards resorption by irradiation ; rather is the result quicker by breaking down and discharge, and consequently quicker healing and less scar formation.

(b) *Tuberculosis of the Bones and Joints.*

Equally good effects are recorded in cases of tuberculosis of the bones and joints. The smaller the children, the more frequent are the occurrences of lighter forms of articular tuberculosis (such as spina ventosa, tuberculosis of the smaller joints, of the carpus or tarsus, ribs, skull, and so forth), the more numerous the foci of disease, and the better are the prospects of cure. Healing takes place often with astonishingly small scars and, even where extensive destruction of bones or joints has occurred, movement is afterwards unimpaired to the smallest degree.*

Tuberculosis of the joints accompanied by sinuses, on the other hand, is often refractory.

Ordinary surgical procedure must not be neglected, particularly immobilization of the affected parts. The process of healing may be accelerated by puncture, drainage of abscesses, and the adjustment of displaced bones

It is difficult to state definite times necessary for cure, but irradiation treatment combined with minor surgery is decisively more advantageous than major surgical procedure or spontaneous

*Birk and Schall.

cure.* Riedel† recommends combined treatment with the quartz and Sollux lamps.

(c) *Tuberculosis of the Skin.*

Beneficial results are reported, and have been observed by myself from irradiation treatment of tuberculosis of the skin. With lichen scrophulosus, intensive radiations leading to desquamation of the upper diseased epidermal layers gives excellent results. In scrofuloderma the action is less rapid ; some months are usually necessary for successful treatment. Cold abscesses in the skin, after drainage by incision, heal in a few weeks (Birk and Schall).

These forms of tuberculosis in children, in which spontaneous healing is itself not uncommon, are certainly the most fruitful field for artificial Alpine Sun quartz lamp treatment.

B. TUBERCULOSIS OF THE INTERNAL ORGANS.

(a) *Peritonitis tuberculosa.*

All writers agree in stating that the effects of artificial Alpine Sun treatment are very favourable in cases of abdominal tuberculosis. The serous form can always be cured by this method without operation, and very satisfactory results, far superior to those from surgery or drugs, have also been achieved in the fibrino-plastic form, even when complicated by adhesions of the omentum and intestines, and by caseo-purulent and hardened tubercular swellings.

From the work on infantile peritonitis tuberculosa by Professor Finkelstein and myself, describing the experiences of the past ten years among the numerous cases of this disease treated in the Kaiser und Kaiserin Friedrich Hospital of Berlin, the indubitable superiority of conservative radiation treatment to the local treatment, and the use of medicaments, and (to a limited extent) operative methods formerly practised, is apparent.

During the post-war period, when the artificial Alpine Sun was brought into use, the results achieved in the treatment of tubercular peritonitis were incomparably more successful, in spite of considerably lowered conditions of existence, than before the war, when the quartz lamp was not in use.

The following figures speak for themselves :—In the pre-war

*Hamburger.
†*Strahlentherapie*, vol. xiii., 1922.

period 50% and during the war 35% of all cases of tubercular peritonitis were treated successfully, while in the post-war period good results were reached in 85%.

From a further comparison of the same material, it appears that the percentages of favourable results obtained by means of artificial Alpine Sun treatment, soft soap treatment, and by operation, were 70, 33, and 43 respectively. " It is probable that the results of laparotomy would have been more favourable, if more children had been operated upon ; this, however, could only have been achieved by including cases which were curable by conservative methods, so that operation would have been resorted to unnecessarily. But in no event would the net results of surgical treatment have surpassed those obtained by the conservative method."

Given adequate nursing and nourishment, and the possibility of prolonged fresh-air treatment, prognosis in the serous form of peritonitis tuberculosa is most favourable. The addition of radiation treatment may accelerate the cure, and may also " give a turn in the right direction in some of the more refractory cases," but it is not so urgently indicated in this as in the adhesive form.

As regards the latter, the introduction of systematic radiation with natural or artificial light--in conjunction of course with good food, proper attention, and superabundance of fresh air—constitutes a considerable advance. The longer the standing of the disease the more difficult to influence favourably. The results of quartz lamp treatment seem to be best in acute cases.

On the other hand, it does not seem possible to secure beneficial results from irradiation in the ulcerated form of the disease, tuberculosis of the bowels, which is difficult to separate clinically from other forms.

Pfefferkorn, describing experiences in the Halle Medical Clinic, expresses himself on similar lines ; also Marchionini, from results at the Leipzig Children's Clinic ; likewise Gerstenberger and Spencer. From the accounts by Selma Meyer of experiences in treating peritonitis tuberculosa at the Berlin Children's Clinic, from 40–50% of the cases treated exclusively by radiation were cured.

Light treatment of the disease is decidedly preferable to internal and surgical methods. The pain generally diminishes very rapidly, and the patient's general condition improves, even in cases not completely curable.

The radiation should be continued for a whole year if possible, even if improvement is noted much earlier, since relapses may otherwise occur years after a cure has been obtained.

(b) Hilus Tuberculosis.

Reports on successful results of irradiation treatment of hilus tuberculosis are not unanimous.   Where this occurred as a subsidiary complaint, no effect from light treatment could be established.   In my own practice I also have failed to ascertain any definite effects from the quartz light treatment.   On the other hand, it is an excellent tonic and, in conjunction with good nursing and nourishment, sound hygienic conditions, and plenty of air and sun, is well suited to increase the body's powers of fighting the infection ; and this is particularly true during the sunless winter months.

C. Pulmonary Tuberculosis.

Tuberculosis pulmonum is another condition in which there is little agreement among authors as to the successes obtainable by the use of the quartz lamp.   The difficulties of judging results are particularly great in this disease, owing to its manifold forms, variable course and the impossibility of obtaining even passably certain data for prognosis by means of X-ray and clinical examination.   Direct action by the rays on the tubercle bacilli can hardly be assumed owing to their limited penetration.   Advanced processes of the lungs with a tendency towards breaking down are unsuitable for radiation treatment ; in any event, no therapeutic success of any kind can be expected in such cases.

The critical treatise of E. Mayer, in which little importance is ascribed to the quartz lamp in comparison with natural sunlight for treating surgical tuberculosis, describes its action in pulmonary tuberculosis as at best that of a stimulant.   On the other hand, Marchionini found at the Leipzig Children's Clinic that slight and moderate cases of pulmonary tuberculosis were always generally, and often physically, benefited, whilst only in severe cases was irradiation unsuccessful.   Gödde excludes severe and febrile cases from radiation treatment, holding its use dangerous ; Birk and Schall, on the contrary, have never seen harm of any sort, including hæmorrhage, from irradiation of children suffering from pulmonary tuberculosis.   None the less, it is in my opinion inadvisable to administer actinotherapy to children in acute stages, above all to those in whom the state of the lungs causes high and continuous fever.

In connection with the small therapeutic success obtainable from radiation in disseminated human tuberculosis of the organs, mention may be made of Hase's experiments on guinea pigs. Of twelve animals infected with tuberculosis, six were radiated, the others untreated ; no effect on the specific process could be established. In view of the slight penetration of the rays this could hardly have been expected.

In " serous effusions of the pleural cavity " radiations are recommended as promising success. Mulierowna states that 40 to 50 treatments are generally sufficient to effect a cure ; on account of the length of the time required, I should consider irradiation alone inferior to the method which I have found most suitable in such cases (hot packs, radiant heat, salicylates without para- centesis) ; although decidedly useful as an adjuvant.

In all cases, however, even if no objective improvement occurs, and no increase in weight is registered, subjective improvement is noticed fairly regularly.

The full use of the tonic action of actinotherapy to assist the usual internal treatment would appear, therefore, worth investiga tion and prescription, even in the two last-named forms of tuberculosis.

D. Children with Positive Pirquet-Reaction.

If it is realized that a positive Pirquet-reaction is not evidence of active tuberculosis, but only a sign that the child has at some time been infected by the disease, the following comments may be made on the relative frequency of this positive result :—

1. If the condition of the organs, observed over a reasonable period, remains negative, the tuberculous infection has not gone further than the primary affection or a small glandular focus (throat, bronchial, or mesenteric gland), and is probably on the way to healing or already cured.

Irradiation is not necessary in such cases, unless the children are run-down, or living under adverse conditions, such as unhealthy surroundings or fresh possibilities of infection in the family.

2. If after some time symptoms present themselves which could possibly be connected with tuberculous infection, a course of artificial Alpine Sun irradiation is advisable, even when there

appears no urgent reason for connecting the symptoms with the disease ; and the younger the child, the more strongly is the treatment indicated.

In both cases the effect of the artificial Alpine Sun may be conceived as that of an excellent tonic, not only for use in the sunless months, but the whole year through ; this on account of the very great practical difficulty of carrying out irradiation during the summer with natural sunlight, owing to its uncertainty and the difficulties of exact dosage.

As regards the duration of irradiation treatment, the course should not be too short, if in addition to improvement in the general condition and pronounced successful results a prolonged after-effect is desired. It happens only too frequently that when irradiation, administered for three or four weeks, has been discontinued owing to good and apparently sufficient results, the children have relapsed after a short time. On this account I recommend two to three months as a minimum period for treatment in such cases.

4. INFANTILE ERYSIPELAS.

There are numerous accounts dealing with successes from radiation in adult cases, and Hedwig Schenk-Popp reports good results in infantile cases at the Freiburg Children's Clinic. In the cases reported, the disease spread on the first day, was checked on the second, and on the third began to recede. Pétenyi obtained identical results in 14 cases, only two of which terminated fatally, and Czepa has made similar observations. On the other hand, Hamburger's statement to the effect that of 8 children treated for erysipelas by irradiation at the Berlin Children's Clinic, six died, and that only two recovered—the one after a fortnight's treatment, and the other after three weeks—is not very encouraging.

Birk and Schall were also unable to trace any results in quartz lamp radiation in erysipelas ; Weltring, on the other hand, believes that " indubitable benefit " results and recommends intensive radiations. Brunauer gives a new technique for erysipelas, tested on 14 cases : at a distance of 20 inches, only the white area surrounding the erysipelatous patch is irradiated (commencing with one minute and increasing by one-half) ; the erysipelas itself, and the healthy skin, being covered. In most cases, a sharp rise of temperature occurs after one or two irradiations ; and cure after four to five treatments. The basis of this success is ascribed to primary injury of the ferments in the cells, thus checking the conditions in the erysipelatous area which favour an extension oɪ the disease.

5. AFFECTIONS OF THE UMBILICUS, LOCAL AND PROGRESSIVE DISCHARGES.

Hedwig Schenk-Popp also reports favourable results in the treatment of other infantile diseases, such as affections of the umbilicus, and progressive discharges of pus. Weltring obtained favourable results in acute lymphadenitis by intensive local radiation.

6. SKIN DISEASES : ECZEMA.

Since it has been proved that lartificia Alpine Sun light possesses bactericidal properties, its use in parasitic diseases, particularly of the skin is justifiably recommended. Satisfactory results are claimed in various cases of eczema accompanied by severe itching.

In pruriginous forms, also, relief of irritation is obtained in most cases by radiation. Mosse, of the Berlin Children's Clinic, recommends the following course for treatment of neurogenous eczema :—After all areas not affected by the disease have been covered (by garments, or protective ointment in the immediate margins), the skin is irradiated twenty to twenty-five minutes at a distance of 10 inches ; after subsidence of the inflammation a second irradiation follows about eight to ten days later, and so forth. In most cases three to four treatments are sufficient for cure ; this technique naturally has no effect on the child's constitution.

Particularly suitable subjects for quartz light therapy are the chronic, infiltrated cases of infantile eczema, as a rule the consequence of eczema in babyhood, which seriously affect the skin and general condition during early years up to school age. Birk and Schall recommend, " to soften the skin," preliminary ointment treatment (first " desquamative paste," then tar and zinc ointment) and daily irradiation, which must be continued after healing is established, accompanied by the application of some skin cream. My own experiences are that dry zinc painting in addition to irradiation is particularly useful, to be combined when severe inflammation is present with moist bandages (acetic Fuller's earth) and preceding irradiation if necessary. It is self-evident that the child must be prevented from scratching. Even in the pruriginous forms irradiation usually gives certain and speedy alleviation from the itching.

Gralka reports favourable results in treating " pemphigus neonatorum." My own experiences in this condition are not sufficiently conclusive to be cited in either sense. The favourable results reported by Michaelis and Weltring in " lichen strophulus infantum " and " impetigo contagiosa " have been also observed by myself.

As to the action of the quartz lamp on the skin, I do not think there is much difference between its effects upon adults and upon children. I therefore refer the reader to the later chapters of this book, dealing with skin diseases.

7.   WHOOPING COUGH.

Some authors recommend artificial Alpine Sun treatment for whooping cough, some direct radiation of the pharynx, and some ascribe to it a prophylactic effect. Hamburger was unable to endorse these recommendations, but in view of the fact that it is often possible in long-standing cases to reduce the severity of the attacks by influencing the patient's mental condition, this may account for the beneficial effects observed by some writers. This assumption of a purely psychological action, which is held by Schotten as well as myself, is doubted by Laqueur, according to whom experience shows that " the quartz lamp has a certain anti-infectious property in many infectious diseases (tuberculosis, erysipelas, furunculosis)." The clinical establishment of indubitable success in irradiated cases of whooping cough, where the disease had been positively diagnosed in the *stadium incremendi*, and where psychological effects did not come into question, would be more convincing than this theoretical consideration. Such cases as this are unfortunately absent from among those described by Schotten ; in all, with one exception, the whooping cough was already of many weeks' standing, and might well, therefore, have passed its crisis. I therefore subjoin brief notes on cases of this kind in my own experience :—

In one case a striking decrease in the night attacks after the beginning of irradiation was established, just as diagnosis had been positively made ; in the course of two days these diminished from six to four, then to two attacks, and then to one during the night ; at the same time, the vomiting, which, up to then, had been very severe, disappeared. Not always are cases treated thus early by irradiation characterized by such prompt success, but if in others the number of attacks did not decrease so speedily, the severity of the individual paroxysms was markedly diminished, their duration shortened, and the subsequent vomiting less frequent, until it disappeared altogether.

When it is considered that this implies beginning treatment at a time when, according to the clinical nature of whooping cough, increase in the severity of the disease must be expected ; and further, that psychological action can as yet be hardly possible, it is only reasonable to suppose that the artificial Alpine Sun action in whooping cough is certainly rather more than a mere tonic and non-specific suggestion. I therefore do not hesitate to recommend its use when opportune, although the question whether its action is specific and assured still requires further confirmatory experiment. The suggestion of Birk and Schall that the apparent successes of quartz light therapy in whooping cough have not stood up to later tests is one which, as the result of numerous inquiries, I cannot confirm ; and I have the impression that the extreme conservatism formerly existent regarding the use of mercury vapour quartz light in this disease is unjustified. Woodward reports good effects following the simultaneous use of quartz light irradiation and pertussis vaccine ; early treatment gave the best results.

The prophylactic effect claimed by some authors is highly improbable. Infection in whooping cough occurs, of course, by means of the particularly virulent secretion, usually in the catarrhal stage, during which the complaint is hardly ever recognized as such, although it occasionally takes place also at the commencement of the paroxysmal stage. After that the danger of infection rapidly decreases and is very slight—if present at all—during the stage of decline. It follows that the danger zone, owing to the manner of infection, is limited to a distance of about 7 feet (2 metres). Contact with a whooping cough patient without development of the infection does not therefore prove very much.

8. Chorea, Enuresis, Asthma, Nervous Disorders.

As regards the successful results reported by various writers in a number of other disorders which may be looked upon as connected with existent neuropathic constitution, it is in my opinion, just as with adults, possible to obtain successes in pediatrics by means of suggestion. It is, of course, presupposed that the children are of sufficient growth to be responsive to suggestion. The successes achieved in the treatment of enuresis, asthma, chorea, and certain nervous troubles, can be explained in this way. If, therefore, other methods fail, I should hold artificial Alpine Sun irradiation advisable, and promising possible success. It is particularly suitable for the suggestive treatment of nervous disorders, the more so because owing to its stimulative effect upon the skin functions, and thus on the circulation, unmistakable improvement of the patient's general condition results in every case, so that the patient is readily supposed to believe that the complaint from which he suffers has also been favourably affected. This view of the radiation treatment as a non-specific remedy of a suggestive character has been endorsed by Hamburger, Birk and Schall, and others.

9. Blood Diseases (Anaemia, etc.) in Childhood.

In blood disorders there is, in my opinion, scarcely any appreciable difference between children and adult patients. Despite the fact that the somewhat optimistic expectations which were entertained when the artificial Alpine Sun method was first applied to them have not been completely fulfilled, it is nevertheless a fact that improvement, as shown, for instance, by hæmoglobin content, erythrocytes count and colour index, have been brought about, if to a less extent than by natural sunlight treatment.

Koenigsfeld could not trace any effect on the erythrocytes and hæmoglobin, but observed after the first irradiations a comparative increase in polynuclear, and often of the mononuclear leucocytes, then simultaneous increase of the lymphocytes and eosinophiles, usually accompanied by a steep drop in the polynuclear and a slow decrease in the large mononuclear cells. After further irradiations the blood count returned to normal ; only a certain eosinophilia usually remained.

Koopmann writes in the same sense. Kopits observed in most cases, in addition to increase of hæmoglobin content, of the colour

indices and of erythrocytes count, a right-hand shift with decrease
of neutrophil cells and increase of eosinophils, monocytes and
lymphocytes ; *i.e.*, a blood condition which is particularly advantageous in resisting tuberculosis. Schoop, whose observations
agree with the Romberg school, has also established this right-
hand shift in Schilling's blood cell-values ; but has the impression
that it is even more evident after local protein shock doses than
after general irradiations.

Margarete Levy found from experiments on rats and mice that
protracted irradiations led to intensive hyperæmia, perivascular
round cell filtrations, and extensive necroses of the liver. When
previous experimental injury to this organ has been conducted,
subsequent irradiation does not promote processes of regeneration,
but checks them. In cases of injury to the liver parenchyma, it
follows that ultra-violet therapy is not applicable ; it favours
erythropoiesis and leucopoiesis, and the removal of pathological
erythrocytes, and is therefore indicated in cases of severe anæmia,
but not in such blood diseases as are accompanied by increased
erythropoiesis and leucopoiesis (leucæmia).

Blood pressure can be affected by quartz lamp treatment during
childhood also. Alice Meyer reports that 60 minutes' treatment
gives an average decrease of blood pressure amounting to 10–8 mm.
Hg. Königsfeld could not effect such large decreases ; his experience was of drops ranging from 2–8 mm. ; protracted irradiation
occasionally caused slight increases.

10. WEAKNESS AND EXHAUSTION.

Particularly suitable for irradiation treatment are conditions of
weakness and exhaustion in childhood, such as frequently occur
after operations and exhausting diseases, and to which delicate
children brought up in large towns are often liable without particular cause. The artificial Alpine Sun treatment has achieved
splendid successes in this respect, and these can be materially
enhanced if the treatment is combined with a change of surroundings.

The appetite soon improves, the circulation is stimulated, and
the change brought about in the child's outlook and general
condition is sometimes surprisingly rapid. Increase in weight
occurs, and irradiation administered over a sufficient period soon
gives markedly increased resistance to infection.

Birk and Schall also report that they have established a most favourable " tonic " action on school children, who are found from experience to be very prone to weakness during the second half of the winter, through increase of school work on the one hand and lack of sunlight on the other. Similar observations were made at the Würzburg Children's Clinic.

II. TECHNIQUE.

1. GENERAL IRRADIATIONS.

As regards actinotherapy technique, we must distinguish between general and local radiations, the latter being applied when only local effects are required.

With the exception of skin diseases, I have made little use of local radiations, and, generally speaking, I recommend general radiation for children. This also applies when it is required to treat localized tuberculous foci and morbid processes, as, simultaneously with the local effect produced, the rays exercise a favourable influence upon the general condition.

Treatment should be started by radiations lasting 3–5 minutes, at 30–40 inches distance, the front and back each being exposed for half this time (*i.e.*, $1\frac{1}{2}$–$2\frac{1}{2}$ minutes each).

Provided that special precautions are taken in the case of babies and very young children, and that in each instance the reaction is carefully watched, each consecutive session should be prolonged by 3 minutes until a maximum of 30 minutes has been reached, at the same distance throughout.

If excessive irritation of the skin occurs, it is advisable to let this subside and to recommence with shorter exposures.

Treatment should be applied three times a week.

By proceeding along these lines, it is usually possible to obtain the desired therapeutic effect without having recourse to increase in the number of weekly radiations, or shortening the distance. In the last two measures we have effective methods of increasing the intensity of treatment, in such rare cases as necessitates this ; due precaution should be observed. Longer exposures are not as a rule necessary.

A modified form of general irradiations has been recently recommended by the Tübingen Children's Clinic ; the distance is shortened to 24 inches, and the dosage regulated according to whether a quick effect is required (as in rickets and tetany) or a treatment extending over a long period (as in tuberculosis). In the latter case treatment is given only three times in the week, commencing with six minutes (three each on front and back), increased at each treatment by one minute on each side, until in the fifth week treatment of both front and back has reached fifteen minutes or half-an-hour together ; this amount is maintained for a fortnight, after which treatment is intermitted for another two weeks, recommencing again with the initial dose.

In the former case, however, a commencement is made with three minutes on front and back at a constant distance of 24 inches ; increased by one minute on each side daily until reddening of the skin persists until the next day, at which point treatment is intermitted until the reaction subsides and resumed with the last dosage employed ; the maximum period of the treatment is 30 minutes, at which point it is usually possible to change from daily to treatment three times weekly, owing to pronounced subsidence of the rickety symptoms in the interim. If the irradiations are prophylactic only, for example, for preventing rickets, treatment is given from the commencement three times a week only, using the same technique.

I am accustomed to administer general irradiations with the lamp at 30 to 40 inches distance, and see no urgent reason for decreasing this to 24, since at this latter distance there is always the possibility of injury or powerful reaction with very delicate children. It is also my rule not to interrupt a treatment once commenced, but if possible to carry it through without intermission until the desired results are achieved ; if a break arises from external causes, treatment is resumed at a half or two-thirds of the dose last given, and only in cases of long intermission do I recommence at the original dose. Otherwise, I have long been accustomed to differentiating between treatment daily and three times weekly ; if quick action is required, daily radiations are given, as in rickets, tetany, whooping cough ; if a more protracted effect is concerned, as in tuberculosis, it is sufficient to give treatment three times weekly ; but in these cases it appears to me advisable for better and speedier action to begin at first with daily irradiations, until doses are reached at which one can conceive of certain results (*i.e.*, about fifteen minutes), and only then to change over to three times weekly.

Whether sensitizing dye-stuffs (*e.g.*, eosin) may be used to intensify the light action is an important question which requires further investigation. Gassul injected white mice, before irradiation, with a half to a quarter of a Pravaz syringeful of a 1% sterile aqueous eosin solution, and found much stronger ultra-violet effects in these sensitized animals than in the controls.

György and Gottlieb confirm this sensitizing action on rachitic infants to whom 0·1 eosin was administered daily by the mouth. The duration of treatment could be greatly diminished (even to half of the customary time). Käthe Pilling and Hottinger write in the same sense.

2. LOCAL IRRADIATION.

Local irradiations are indicated in certain dermatological affections to which children are liable, and should be carried out according to the instructions given by Bach. The surroundings of the affected areas must be suitably protected against the rays, or a suitable small diaphragm opening chosen ; the lamp kept at a distance of 20 inches, and the duration of each treatment extended as described above, *i.e.*, by three minutes each time, until the desired erythema dose is reached. The maximum duration of half-an-hour need not in most instances be exceeded.

If local irradiation is conducted along lines such as these, there is no likelihood of any injuries from their application, and no risk even in treating babies and premature infants.

A larger dose (irradiation lasting 15 to 20 minutes) is recommended by Birk and Schall in the case of certain nervous troubles for which no organic cause can be found (pains in head and back, " stitch " in the side, stomach ache, and so forth) given on an area about the size of the palm of the hand over the painful spot, protecting the remaining skin ; they have observed prompt effect on the pain coupled with reddening of the irradiated areas extending for some days. In this connection attention is drawn to the method of local irradiation described in Section 4 (Erysipelas) and 6 (Neurogenous Eczema) above. Local irradiation, like general, can therefore act well by suggestion.

Liebermeister, who obtained speedy and lasting cure in a case of tuberculous peritonitis through an inadvertent over-powerful irradiation, recommends restricted local irritation doses, in which an area of 4–6 inches diameter is given an erythema dose, and the next treatment given only after subsidence of the reaction. He and Schoop have had good results thus in treating tuberculous peritonitis, lymphomata, and also in tuberculosis of other organs.

3. PRECAUTIONS.

It is, of course, understood that the quartz lamp should only be used by a qualified practitioner or under his direction. If this is true in a general way, it is especially so where children are concerned.

By way of conclusion, I should like to state that, from my experience, the desired effects can be obtained by the use of the artificial Alpine Sun without other lamps, although this can of course be supplemented by the Sollux Lamp or Hagemann Ring.

Special emphasis may again be laid on the importance of irradiating babies and delicate little children in a thoroughly warmed room, so as to prevent colds ; in thus warming the treatment room, particularly at the changes of the year, simultaneous irradiation with the Sollux lamp or other heating lamp is very serviceable ; care must, of course, be taken not to overheat the children, which can easily be managed by regulation of the distance. Stress must also be laid on avoiding chills, after the irradiation ; according to Weltring, this is done at the Würzburg Children's Clinic by dry-rubbing after treatment and then a stay of 10 to 15 minutes in another well-warmed room.

The irritating effect of combustion gases on the respiratory tract, assumed by Birk and Schall, has not been confirmed by the writer, whose experience agrees with that of Weltring in this regard. Catarrh of the upper air-passages never occurred as a consequence of irradiation when the precautions mentioned above were observed, but did so occasionally if these were omitted.

Chicken-pox does not constitute a contra-indication for irradiation ; on the other hand, it is not an indication. Sack, who, during an epidemic of chicken-pox, observed a particularly severe case of this disease in a child previously irradiated with the quartz lamp, assumed that some connection existed between the severity of the attack and the irradiation, in the sense of a sensitizing of the skin, and quickening of the eruptive process. Rohrböck reports the case of one unfortunate child which was strongly attacked on parts of the skin previously irradiated, as compared with other areas of the body, on which the chicken-pox eruptions were sparse.

Reiche, on the other hand, who had twenty cases irradiated before or during the eruptive stage of chicken-pox, could not trace any effects of irradiation ; an observation which I was also able to make on a similar number of cases at my clinic during an epidemic of chicken-pox.

Amongst other harmful results from quartz lamp irradiation, dermitides are sometimes observed as the result of incautious over-dosage ; the occurrence of a mild erythema cannot be so classed, and it is indeed often enough aimed at, particularly in local irradiation. Stronger irritation, accompanied by œdematous swelling, possibly leading to blistering, is, however, a condition which should in any case be avoided, particularly in infants and babies, even although their course does not usually differ from similar skin-irritation arising from other causes.

The isolated instances quoted by Faber and Dotzel, who observed albuminuria of short duration after irradiation erythema, require a somewhat cautious acceptance ; the latter writer does not indeed consider that any connection exists between the condition and the irradiation. In one case, quoted by Römer, a miliary outbreak occurred after artificial Alpine Sun irradiation ; in another, quoted by Austgen, a scarlatinoid exanthem with large lamellar exfoliation occurred after a single short irradiation ; in another, after five minutes irradiation at 20 inches distance of a case of impetigo, pulmonary œdema, accompanied by cessation of heart and respiration, occurred four hours later ; when this condition had subsided the child remained comatose for two days longer. In yet another case, quoted by Röseler, after irradiation of a torpid ulcer on the back of the hand (ten minutes at 4 inches distance), severe vesicular dermatitis occurred involving both hands, the face, throat, and the membrane of the mouth, which, however, healed without scars, leaving heavy pigmentation and increased sensitivity to light.

These cases may in part be due to coincident occurrence of the conditions mentioned with the irradiations, in part they can be ascribed to over-strong dosage. In any case the number of injuries from irradiation reported from the medical profession, in which careful and correct dosage may be presumed, is extraordinarily small, particularly when it is remembered how often quartz light is at present used. The majority of actinotherapists, despite extensive practice, have hardly been able to observe cases in their own experience in which harmful effects could be assumed.

It may well be otherwise if quartz light treatments are carried out by laymen and the dosage not suited to the individual peculiarity of the child treated ; of harmful results so caused, of which reports are very sporadic, we have no further details. Such are perhaps more frequent than one is inclined to suppose ; hence the stringent advice only to conduct irradiation under medical advice and supervision, particularly in childhood.

Summary of Chapter III.

All things considered, quartz light irradiation may be regarded as a very potent addition to the therapeutic armentarium of the pediatrist.

Leaving out of account the fact that, as briefly mentioned above, radiation treatment usually exercises a beneficial effect upon the general condition, a condensed summary follows of those diseases in which there is undoubted benefit from artificial Alpine Sun treatment, together with those in which its effects can be only conditionally recognized.

(1) *Proved Successes of Quartz Light Treatment.*

(*a*) Rickets : A specific action may rightly be assumed in the case of this disease, both as regards certain therapeutic healing of the disease and prophylactic treatment, the results of which are practically certain in preventing its outbreak. Similar good results, based on its anti-rachitic action, are observed in :—

(*b*) Tetany.

(*c*) Surgical Tuberculosis : Of the tuberculous diseases of childhood, this is the most suited for irradiation treatment. Apart from tuberculosis of the joints with sinuses, this applies to all its manifestations, *i.e.,* :—

(1) Lymphadenitis tuberculosa.

(2) Tuberculosis of the bones.

(3) Tuberculosis of the skin.

(*d*) Peritonitis tuberculosa : The exudative forms lend themselves well to treatment, and in the adhesive tumor-like forms, it is superior to the methods formerly used, the results being especially successful in processes of acute origin.

(*e*) Affections of the skin : The benefit of artificial Alpine Sun treatment in these diseases is unmistakable, and the same holds good for (*f*).

(*f*) General weakness and debility in children.

(*g*) Pertussis (Whooping cough) : As the last indication I would mention whooping cough, at the same time emphasizing the fact that this question is still under discussion, since in my experience the effect of ultra-violet goes far beyond that of suggestion, hitherto conceived as its action.

(2) *Successes Not Quite Unexceptionable.*

(*a*) Tuberculosis of the joints : The results from quartz light treatment are not definitely established, especially if the suppuration has found an outlet to the skin. In such cases it is often impossible to register an improvement.

(*b*) Tuberculosis of the hilus, and

(*c*) Pulmonary tuberculosis : In these cases, too, it is difficult to pronounce a definite opinion. In the less advanced stages, the possibility of improvement may be granted. In advanced pulmonary tuberculosis, and the ulcerating forms of tuberculous peritonitis, little result may be expected.

(*d*) Infantile erysipelas.

(*e*) Infections of the umbilicus, local and progressive suppurations, and

(*f*) Anæmia and other infantile blood diseases : In these diseases, also, judgment must be reserved.

A certain effect in chorea, enuresis, asthma, nervous disorders, etc., appears barely conceivable under the limitations mentioned above, only as a measure of suggestion in the case of nervous subjects.

CHAPTER IV.

SKIN DISEASES.

Since the skin is the point where the action of light is developed, its diseases are particularly suitable for light therapy ; and this applies not only to the diseases of the outer skin, but also those of the mucous membranes, as was established by Guthmann of Frankfurt-a-M. on the vaginal mucous membrane. He found that this was twice as resistant to light as the outer skin ; *i.e.*, the vaginal mucous membrane requires double the dosage of light necessary to produce an equal degree of erythema on the skin. In this section, only the diseases of the outer skin are considered, the chapter being based on the text of Keutel's work in the last edition of this book, partly quoted verbatim.

The basis of light action on the skin is stated in Part I. It need only be repeated that erythema therapy with the ultra-violet light of the artificial Alpine Sun quartz lamp, and hyperæmia therapy with the luminous heat rays of the Hanovia Sollux lamp come into consideration. In this section we shall only treat of ultra-violet therapy, so far as no express reference is made to hyperæmia treatment.

Dermatomycoses (Trichophytosis superficialis, Pityriasis rosea et versicolor, Eczema marginatum, Erythrasma).

In these dermatomycoses, where the fungi are deposited on or in the outermost layers of the skin, there is without doubt direct destruction of the fungoid elements through ultra-violet irradiation. On account of the inflammatory reaction, by which the uppermost layers of the epidermis throughout the irradiated area are completely shed, the fungi are also removed by purely mechanical processes, so that the first force of the disease is broken and cure results. It is, however, advisable, in order to prevent relapses, to continue irradiation as long as possible.

Schindler* observed that " even with protracted irradiation erythema never results, if the skin has been plentifully painted with silver nitrate immediately after the commencement of the

---

*Die Behandlung von Dermatosen mit Quartz-Lichtbestrahlungen bei gleichzeitiger Einwirkung von 5% igem Argt. Nitr. spiritus (70%), *Dts. med. Wochenschrift*, 1920, No. 5.

treatment. The rays can only penetrate to the skin and be absorbed so long as the silver nitrate is not completely decomposed. With increasing blackening of the skin—which begins very soon— as soon as the silver chloride has separated out, no more rays penetrate. Avoidance of an erythema is a great boon to the patients. The deep-reaching softening and resorbent action can therefore only be explained through the liberation of nitric acid, which as we know penetrates the tissues deeply. In a frozen section of skin from the back of a white guinea pig, it could be clearly seen that the separated silver was deposited in the horny cells, and therefore quite superficially. The silver cannot therefore play any part in the deep action."

According to Finkenrath,* pityriasis lichenoides chronica can be cured by light alone, one treatment being sufficient provided the dosage be large enough.

FURUNCULOSIS ; CARBUNCLES.

Not only superficial pyodermatitis, but also the more penetrating forms, *e.g.*, furunculosis, respond very favourably to treatment to ultra-violet light. This applies not so much to single boils, which must be treated by the usual methods, as to the massive penetration of the entire surface of the skin with pyogenic bacteria. Here it is possible to use first the bactericidal, then the inflammatory power of ultra-violet rays. Since every boil involves an exudation of staphylococci in its immediate and remote neighbourhood, suitable disinfection of the surrounding area must be conducted. A large proportion of the germs near the surface are killed by the ultra-violet rays, the best disinfectant, whilst those surviving are removed with the peeling of the skin, which takes place far more evenly than by chemical means. Deeper-seated boils, and particularly carbuncles, are checked in their development by intensive radiation, or quickly healed if mature ; the lasting hyperæmia, and apparently still more the anti-bodies formed in the serous influx, causing stoppage of the infection, and isolation of the dead tissue. The inflammatory pain ceases shortly after irradiation. The results obtained by light treatment are identical with those resulting from Bier's passive hyperæmia, and it can be used both in the early stages when suppuration is at its height, and also when

*Dermatol. Zeitschrift, vol. xlvi., 1926.

healing has already commenced. It is, of course, understood that local treatment and vaccine therapy (leucogen, opsinogen, and the staphylococci vaccines of Merk), based on Wright's opsonin theory, should not be neglected.

Seborrhoea, Acne Vulgaris.

Irradiation with ultra-violet rays has a similar action in seborrhœa and acne vulgaris, although results are less rapid. Seborrhoic conditions, however, can only be influenced symptomatically, the radiations having the effect of opening up the pores, and of thus facilitating discharge of the secretion. In the case of acne vulgaris, powerful irradiations are used to open up the sebaceous follicles, and to get rid of the diseased skin by thorough exfoliation. Only milder cases of acne vulgaris which do not exhibit infiltrations of the skin can, however, be treated thus ; such can be practically cured. Severe cases require X-ray treatment in addition.

Freckles.

In extensive cases of freckles, light treatment is recommended as a last resource. Whereas small doses of light, as is known, cause tanning and increase of freckles, powerful radiations have the contrary effect. By means of a very intense light-produced inflammation, strong enough to lead to two or even three peelings of the skin, so that the entire epidermis, together with the pigmented epithelial layer is removed, it is in some cases possible to get rid of this form of pigmentation for good. It is, however, often necessary to reckon with the possibility of a relapse, and to use great care in giving a prognosis. Careful after-treatment by means of cooling paste and powder, which will result in the disappearance of the inflammation in a few days, is of course necessary.

This photogenic inflammation not only causes exfoliation of the outer layers of the skin at the local foci, but also increases the circulation in it. The cellular elements of the blood, erythrocytes, leucocytes, etc., accumulate in the dilated lymph spaces, and also in the intercellular spaces. Owing to the close contact with the tissue-forming cells the red corpuscles are deprived of their oxygen which is then passed on to the cells and distributed. Hence, in consequence of the direct action of the ultra-violet rays, combined with an increase of carbonic acid, greatly intensified metabolism takes place, not only in each separate cell, but throughout the entire tissue. I am inclined to define the changes so produced in the chemical structure of the tissue, whose oxidizing power is augmented by the added hæmoglobin and erythrocytes, as a kind of readjustment of the tissue.

DISEASES OF THE HAIR AND SCALP.

(Alopecia areata, and loss of hair after a skin or generalized disease.)

The improved nutrition of the skin caused thereby is an additional therapeutic effect of treatment with ultra-violet rays, of which special use can be made in treating various diseases of the hair and the scalp. A favourable result of light treatment is noticeable in every case where temporary suspension of function of the hair papillæ is concerned, i.e., whenever the latter, though completely intact, do not form any more hair substance. This applies specially in alopecia areata. All that is needed to stimulate the hair papillæ to renewed activity is to supply them with better nutrition by means of intense stimulation. This can be done easily, and in a manner most convenient to the patient, by irradiation ; which, as regards alopecia areata, is the method of choice. The length of time the condition has lasted is naturally important as regards the success of the treatment, since in recent cases the inactivity of the hair papillæ has not proceeded so far as in older ones.

In cases of loss of hair consequent upon X-ray treatment, irradiation is equally suitable, under the same proviso. Good results are at least obtainable in all cases where the hair papillæ have not yet been destroyed by the X-rays. Loss of hair accompanying or following local skin disease or generalized illness, e.g. typhoid fever, influenza, anæmia, etc., is merely a symptom of general malnutrition, or else the result of a toxic action upon the papillæ, and may disappear without treatment once the causes have been removed. It is, however, obvious from what has been said that healing will be considerably accelerated by improved nutrition of the scalp from intensive irradiation. This may, therefore, always be recommended as a valuable adjuvant, both in the form of local and of general irradiation.

Nagelschmidt described irradiation with the artificial Alpine Sun as definitely effective and comparatively quick in by far the majority of cases of alopecia in its most varied forms, for which it is at present the most certain kind of treatment, and also in many other diseases of the hair. Even if complete cure does not result in every case, improvement is so considerable except in a diminishing minority of cases that the results can usually be described as satisfactory from a cosmetic standpoint. Relapses cannot always be avoided, but can be overcome by ultra-violet irradiation just as easily and certainly as the original disease. To prevent these, Nagelschmidt recommends that even after healing has taken place further irradiations should be given at intervals of a month.

Nagelschmidt further reports that of 104 cases of alopecia areata, 80 were completely cured, 16 showed improvement, whilst 8 remained unaffected.

In 53 cases of seborrhoic alopecia all were cured without exception, most of them after a single radiation. The subjective discomfort ceased, the scales disappeared, lost hair grew again, and the existing hair increased in length.

In lupus erythematosus no new growth of hair occurred on the scars.

In acute primary X-ray alopecia, if not complicated by serious dermatitis, and in syphilis, so far as the skin has not been destroyed by scars, the prognosis is good. The course of the healing process is accelerated by light treatment.

Nagelschmidt's technique is to irradiate from ten to twenty minutes at a distance of 10 to 12 inches. Healthy skin areas must be adequately protected from exposure. If pains in the scalp or neuralgic discomfort result, he prescribed narcotics and poultices of acetate of alumina or $\frac{1}{2}\%$ resorcin water for twelve or twenty-four hours. If the skin reaction to the radiation is very powerful, it is necessary to await subsidence, and the next irradiation can then ensue three or four weeks later. As soon as the skin is no longer sensitive to light, exposures are gradually prolonged up to a maximum of one hour.

Varicose Ulcer, Bubo, and Pernio Exulcerans.

In the case of ulcus cruris—a complaint which frequently requires months of treatment, and in which the tendency to healing is slight—the action of the chemically acting rays upon the irradiated tissues also produces an enormous increase of the metabolic activity, and this after first augmenting the discharge through active hyperæmia, brings about rapid replacement of the sodden floor of the ulcer by active red granulation, and subsequent speedy regeneration of the skin by stimulating cellular proliferation at the epithelial border. If radiations are applied about twice a week until a distinct reaction occurs, the surrounding portions of the skin also being radiated, healing will be effected within a comparatively short period of time with a firm cicatrix. The same holds good for ulcers arising from bubo and broken chilblains.

Jost* observed decrease of pain after the first irradiation in treating chilblains, especially the ulcerated forms, by the quartz lamp. The most obdurate ulcers dried, forming scabs, and went on to rapid cure. Irradiations were commenced with five minutes at a distance of 12–20 inches, and increased by five minutes at each subsequent treatment. The second exposure took place on the day following the first, later ones every second day. As a rule, five or six sessions were sufficient to effect a cure.

Eczema.

Especially in dealing with the chronic, dry, and squamous forms of eczema, the aim is to evoke active inflammation by means of intensive irradiation leading to an acute stage, and then to treat it as an acute form of the disease. If irradiation is given about twice weekly until distinct hyperæmia and desquamation occurs, it certainly appears as though the infiltrations recede more rapidly, and that healing takes place much earlier than by using medicaments alone. Keutel advises against irradiation of acute eczema, since its use not only does not lead to improvement but even to a great aggravation of the disease. Hence, it is also necessary in treating chronic forms, after having evoked an acute stage by irradiation, to alleviate the irritation each time by milder treatment. When this subsides the eczema often shows considerable improvement, or is even cured altogether. This loosening of tissue, which, as it were, prepares the ground for other methods of treatment, is of marked benefit in one kind of chronic eczema, viz., lichen chronicus simplex, which then responds more freely to subsequent ointment and X-ray treatment. The increased circulation brought about by irradiation is not, however, limited to the

---

*Die Behandlung der Frostbeulen mit Quecksilberquarzlicht (" The Treatment of Chilblains by the Mercury Quartz Lamp "), *Schweizer Medizinische Wochenschrift*, No. 52, 1920.

local focus, but affects its surroundings as well, and—if the whole body is exposed to the rays—the entire system, as is shown by the increase in erythrocytes and hæmoglobin, with rise in the temperature of the skin and simultaneous decrease of internal temperature ; general effects, which are achieved by influencing the functions of the skin. These skin functions are of great importance in the modern conception, since according to Bloch the skin has the power of producing immunizing substances (esophylaxis), which special activity of the skin is greatly increased by irradiation.

Irradiation accompanied by simultaneous painting of the skin with *argt spiritus* has, according to Schindler, proved of special value in many dry forms of eczema, in which previous treatment with ointment and quartz light had had little effect. This also applied in perioral eczema and other highly irritating intertriginous forms of eczema on the upper thigh. After two irradiations the irritation ceased. Several hypertrophic forms of sycosis were also cured by this treatment. The treatment of chronic infiltrated eczema with ultra-violet light, recently described by Birk and Schall, seems to offer particularly good prospects. It consists in preliminary treatment with ointments and more prolonged after-treatment under the artificial Alpine Sun.

Neurogenous eczema, located chiefly in the bends of knee and elbow, was successfully treated by Mosse* using quartz light as follows :—

The diseased skin areas were irradiated at about 10 inches distance, for 20–30 minutes, the non-affected areas having been well covered. During the days following irradiation intense reddening developed on the areas treated, coupled with swelling, which was followed by shedding of the entire outer layers of the epidermis. After eight to ten days all reactive symptoms have usually subsided and the practitioner can proceed to the next irradiation. In the majority of cases 3–4 irradiations suffice for the disappearance of the skin symptoms ; and the irritation usually subsides one or two days after the irradiation. Scrupulous protection of the healthy skin is important, in order to avoid burns, and is best carried out by means of ointment in the immediate neighbourhood of the eczematous patch, and by thick clothing on other parts.

*Deutsche med. Wochenschrift, 1925, No. 51.

PEMPHIGUS VULGARIS AND DERMATITIS HERPETIFORMIS.

The tonic effect of ultra-violet rays upon the whole system has been utilized with particular success for treating such skin diseases as are accompanied by certain internal complications which are still unexplained. Thus, it may be stated regarding pemphigus vulgaris, and dermatitis herpetiformis, which closely resembles it, that their course is undeniably affected in a favourable manner by irradiation with the artificial Alpine Sun quartz lamp. In some instances the results from irradiation therapy are not so good, but in other instances much better than those achieved from arsenic treatment alone. Comparatively good results are obtained by a combination of both methods. To achieve permanent cure, it is imperative to continue irradiation intermittently as long as possible, and in the event of the slightest relapse, to resume it in conjunction with arsenic and with the quinine treatment which has proved so excellent in these conditions.

PSORIASIS VULGARIS.

Many authorities use ultra-violet treatment for the non-elevated diffuse types of psoriasis showing little desquamation. It cannot be denied that distinct improvement sometimes occurs from the inflammatory reaction accompanied by slight serous exudation (analogous to the effects produced by the reducing agents usually employed), from the metabolic stimulation throughout the system, and the consequent favourable effect upon the patient's general condition. On the other hand, it should be remembered that psoriasis sometimes disappears for a time without any treatment, so that it does not follow with absolute certainty that disappearance of the symptoms can be placed to the exclusive credit of the treatment. Many cases, indeed, remain entirely unaffected by the rays, and unfavourable results are sometimes observed, although these again need not be ascribed to irradiation, since they also occur with the application of other methods. Keutel has doubts, however, concerning Linser's statement* that of 100 patients treated by light a considerable proportion were cured without relapses, inasmuch as the occurrence of relapses is one of the features typical of psoriasis, which has been found impossible

*Über die Behandlung der Psoriasis mit ultra-violetten Licht (" The Treatment of Psoriasis by Ultra-Violet Rays,") *Medizinische Klinik*, No. 27, 1915.

to prevent by any known treatment. This view is shared by Jolles,* who recommends general irradiation with the artificial Alpine Sun in conjunction with X-ray treatment of the individual patches in order to strengthen the skin. On the other hand, Kumar† writes that ultra-violet light, particularly recommended by Linser, is often extraordinarily beneficial in psoriasis. The doses to be used must be so strong that a definite inflammatory reaction results. It follows from this that only cases with isolated, few, large foci can be treated by this means.

PRURITUS.

Both the general and local forms of pruritus require symptomatic in addition to radical treatment. Medical science knows many anti-pruritic devices, but these are often ineffective in curing this unpleasant complaint. Since it is mostly due to the irritant effects produced upon the vascular nerves of the skin by certain irritating or toxic substances which are brought thither by the blood, and since intensive application of ultra-violet rays results in improved metabolism throughout the organism, it can be recommended as an adjuvant to the ordinary radical therapy (urticaria interna, pruritus in association with diabetes and liver complaints). Moreover, in senile pruritus—which is generally due to a failure of the normal skin functions—the enhanced blood supply to the tissues resulting from such radiation often produces surprising success after few erythema doses.

ATROPHIES OF PIGMENT, VITILIGO, LEUCODERMA SYPHILITICUM.

For the treatment of skin diseases erythema treatment is more frequently used when the aim is to improve the blood supply of the diseased tissues, and thus secure increased metabolic activity. But when it is intended to remove pigment atrophies, mild irradiation without erythema formation has also been tried as a therapeutic measure. The results obtained are far from satisfactory, although better with vitiligo, in which it is at least possible to bring about a temporary darkening of the skin by extended ultra-violet

*Die Strahlenbehandlung in der Dermatologie (" Irradiation in Dermatology "), *Nederlandsch Tijdschrift voor Geneeskunde*, vol. lxv., Part II., No. 18, 1921.

†*Wien. Klin. Wochenschrift*, 1924, No. 36.

irradiation.   Leucoderma syphiliticum cannot be influenced by therapeutic treatment, and quartz lamp irradiation is also ineffective here, according to Keutel and other writers.

Keutel is also of opinion that other syphilitic skin diseases are unsuitable for ultra-violet treatment ; syphilitic varicose ulcers, among other conditions, being more easily affected unfavourably than otherwise by quartz light.

Since Breiger reported successful results in treating syphilis with quartz light irradiation, the use for and against light therapy in this disease has been described by various authors.   Hesse*, who recommends sunlight treatment in secondary syphilis, holds that the fact that healing processes are activated by light in the most varied acute and chronic stages of syphilis cannot be controverted, and that the subject affected by syphilis can derive the greatest benefit therefrom, coupled with the approved medicaments.

Spiethoff† investigated the effect of ultra-violet rays upon exanthems during the early stages of syphilis, the action of indirect irradiation on the spirochetes, the reactive effect of quartz light on exanthems which have already subsided, and the influence of irradiation on the Wassermann reaction.   From these, there are effects in the sense of a " healing tendency " present, but these natural defensive measures of organism, stimulated and strengthened by irradiation, rarely or never suffice, like the healing efforts of the body when unaided, to overcome the infection.

In contradiction to Breiger, who observed a cure of syphilis by ultra-violet irradiation, Spiethoff states that a " specific " treatment can never be replaced by a " non-specific " stimulation therapy (as he terms it), nor supplemented or assisted by simultaneous light treatment.   He considers, however, that the tonic action of irradiation is indicated when the patient complains of certain general symptoms, such as weakness, etc.

TUBERCULOSIS CUTIS.

Keutel writes :   " The various forms of skin tuberculosis have always proved valuable criteria of the effects of irradiation.   It is easily understood why a particularly strict delimitation of the indications for quartz light treatment has been established in the

*Strahlentherapie, vol. xii., 1921.

†Dermat. Zeitschr, vol. xlvii., 1926.

therapy of lupus. Klingmüller and Halberstädter* proved by numerous experiments that even by Finsen treatment tubercle bacilli located close to the surface are not destroyed. The innate bactericidal properties of the light play therefore no part in the treatment of tuberculosis cutis. The process of healing in the tubercular foci is evoked rather by the inflammatory effect of the rays, and perhaps also by their pigment-producing action. The foci exhibit changes due to the reactive inflammation, which are followed by dilatation and hyperæmia of the arterial vessels and by exudation of a serous character, effecting the entire tuberculous infiltration. The chief aim should therefore be to flood the irradiated tuberculous focus with extravasated serum. By means of this exudation, flooding the diseased tissue, new strength is given to the weakened natural defensive powers of the system against tubercle bacilli, and this new force overcomes the disease in consequence of its protective substances. For the effective treatment of lupus, general radiations should not be omitted in addition to local. The value of such general treatment of lupus patients in the form of light baths is not yet properly appreciated. They have a pronounced beneficial effect on the patient's general condition, owing to the increase in metabolism, but apart from this they also promote the cure of tuberculosis cutis in its various forms in so far as they make the foci more amenable to local treatment, whether this consists in the application of X-rays, ointments, or any other methods. Practical experience has shown that the artificial Alpine Sun irradiation alone, continued to the point of distinct inflammation, decidedly produces beneficial effects upon the lupus patient, but that these effects are inferior to those produced by Finsen light or X-rays. This is also shown by the histological fact that the changes produced are much less deep or extensive than those produced by the other radiological methods mentioned. Treatment by ultra-violet rays can therefore only be described as an adjuvant—although a very effective one—which, combined with other approved methods, guarantees definitely successful results. Preliminary treatment by tuberculin, operation, chemical erosion by ointment, very considerably augments the action of light upon lupus, since the light rays and X-rays can

---

*From Bering, Über die Wirkung violetter und ultravioletter Lichtstrahlen (" The Effect of Violet and Ultra-Violet Rays "), published in the *Medizinische-Naturwissenschaftliches Archiv*, No. 1 (1907), Berlin.

penetrate comparatively deeply once the wound surfaces have been cleansed, and the scab caused by the pyrogallic acid has been cleared away. Hence it is advisable to combine treatment with X-rays and ultra-violet rays in such a manner that a quartz light irradiation should be followed up two or three days later by X-ray treatment, since the latter is especially effective so long as the inflammatory reaction from irradiation is still in evidence. Subject to the precautions mentioned, the superficial variety of lupus, which spreads rather than penetrates, offers best prospects for light treatment, although good results are also obtained in other forms. Skin regeneration occurs in ulcerated forms, while the hypertrophic and verrucous varieties are reduced after being treated by ultra-violet rays exclusively, so that the latter are a valuable adjuvant in their case also ; the more so since by ultra-violet, suitably combined with other approved methods of treatment, a satisfactory cosmetic result may be obtained, the final scar being of neat and delicate tissue."

As far as Keutel's experience goes, the treatment of lupus erythematosus by ultra-violet rays produces no effects whatever.

Jesionek writes in his work, " Die Sonnenlichtbehandlung des Lupus " (" The Insolation Treatment of Lupus "), published in *Strahlentherapie*, vol. ix., No. 1 (1920) :—

" Moreover, in cases of lupus we have observed cures and curative processes which we had to regard as indirectly due to the action of the rays, effected through the medium of the skin, or, as I formerly expressed it, through the pigment, and I am to-day no longer certain with a clear conscience that these may be ascribed solely to the favourable effect of the rays upon the general condition of the patient acting through a non-specific photo-genetic secretion of the basal cells. Further, that I believe I may safely state that the introduction of heliotherapy for our lupus patients—a treatment which, at first calculated exclusively on the pigment-producing property of light—has been a success in that it has not only prevented, in a number of our patients, local relapses, but even relapses of any description which could have been ascribed to tubercular foci still present in the body, and that the healing of superficial lupus foci exposed to the inflammatory action of light, has in general required less time than has been the case without the combination of local and general irradiation. We have also found—and I may here state that we should perhaps regard lupus as an allergic reaction of the skin to endogenous infection—that cutaneous innoculations of tuberculin by the Deycke-Much partial antigen, in tuberculous patients whose skin has acquired a healthy appearance and strong pigmentation from sunbaths, have produced less positive effects than in patients with unpigmented skin of an anæmic and unhealthy appearance ; occasionally, in fact, these innoculations have been negative, not only on pigmented parts of the skin, but also on those parts which had intentionally not been exposed to the pigmenting action of light. We have gained the conviction that the effects of light which are beneficial, objectively considered, are also evident in the case of tuberculosis and lupus, or rather, that they are particularly conspicuous in these cases. We are inclined to believe that this is not only due to the tonic effect of light upon the general power of resistance possessed by the tissues to tubercular toxins, but rather also to specific effects upon the skin tissue in the sense that the latter, under the action of light, loses those properties to which it is due that the pathogenic lodgment of the tubercle bacilli in the skin produces that particular type of tubercular skin disease which we term Lupus."

TECHNIQUE.

So far as the technique of irradiation is not stated in the section on individual diseases, the rules of dosage given in Part I. apply. In all skin diseases, the diseased skin area should in the first place be given local irradiation, but as a rule general irradiation is also indicated as a means of raising the general condition, which is usually lowered. By this again the local condition is not infrequently ameliorated, as Jesionek has demonstrated in the case of lupus. He was even able to cure certain cases of lupus by general irradiation alone when the lupus foci were kept covered from the action of the rays.

SUMMARY.

(a) *Established successes :—*

Dermatomycoses (trichophytia superficialis, pityriasis rosea and versicolor, eczema marginatum, erythrasma).

Furunculosis and Carbuncles.

M

Alopecia areata (loss of hair following skin diseases or general diseases).

Varicose ulcers, bubo, and pernio exulcerans (broken chilblains).

Tuberculosis cutis.

(b) *Results not definitely established :—*

Seborrhœa, acne vulgaris.

Freckles.

Eczema.

Pemphigus vulgaris, dermatitis herpetiformis.

Pruritus.

Psoriasis vulgaris.

Pigment atrophies (vitiligo, leucoderma syphiliticum).

Syphilis.

CHAPTER V.

GYNÆCOLOGY.

THE artificial Alpine Sun quartz lamp has also found manifold uses in gynæcology. Seeing that many abdominal diseases differ only in localization from other diseases (*e.g.*, tuberculosis, sepsis, circulatory disturbances, etc.), it is not surprising that good results follow local and general irradiation administered according to the dosage stated in Part I. According to Guthmann, the vaginal membrane is also suitable for ultra-violet treatment, as already mentioned in the section on skin diseases. According to him, also, the dosage is twice that required for the outer skin.

WOUNDS, GRANULATIONS, ULCERS, AND PRURITUS.

In these external conditions, Heynemann* has established the pronounced bactericidal effects of direct irradiation by ultra-violet rays, although these—as is well known—do not penetrate deeply. He obtained successful results in treating septic wounds (*e.g.*, septic of the abdominal wall following operation, varicose ulcers during pregnancy). Flabby granulations were turned into healthy ones, and the process of healing was accelerated, through destruction of the germs, desiccation of the wound, and stimulation of the healing process. Granulating wounds tolerate powerful irradiations which would be inapplicable, except perhaps after some time, in treating the outer skin or the more easily inflamed parts of the mucous membranes. The same applies to ulcers in cases of prolapse. Van de Velde† reports successful results in cases of ulcers, prolapse, varicose ulcers, certain eczematous diseases of the labiæ, the perineum, the regions of the anus and the mons veneris, and, above all, in cases of pustular inflammations.

Heynemann‡ states that pruritus vulvæ is also suitable for quartz light irradiation, and Van de Velde, Fromme, and Rotschuh

*Uber Verwendug der Ultravioletten Strahlen in der Gynäkologie und den Einfluss dieser und anderer Strahlen auf Bakterien ("On the Use of the Ultra-Violet Rays in Gynæcology, and the Effects of these and other Rays upon Bacteria.")

†*Zentralblatt für Gynäkologie*, No. 19, 1915.

‡*Address delivered before the Freie Vereinigung Mitteldeutscher Gynäkologen, on May 17th*, 1914.

have endorsed his view. On the other hand, O. Schlein* reports that irradiation proved ineffective in most cases. He recommends X-ray treatment for pruritus.

Cases due to nervous irritability or to the irritant effect of leukorrhœa upon the genital organs practically always benefit from the application of the artificial Alpine Sun treatment. Those, however, which are caused by metabolic disturbances (*e.g.* diabetes, gout) can be effectively dealt with only by appropriate treatment of the original disease.

DISEASES OF THE VAGINA AND CERVIX.

Heynemann, Wagner, Van de Velde, and F. M. Meyer have successfully used the artificial Alpine Sun quartz lamp in dealing with vaginal catarrhs, and erosions of the cervix. Van de Velde observed satisfactory results in cases of obdurate, non-malignant erosions of the cervix, and of chronic vaginitis, and effected a permanent cure of a case of tuberculosis of the vaginal cervix by means of irradiation. Wagner cured erosions of the cervix, which had obstinately resisted all other treatment, after six radiations, producing a firm epithelium. During each session first the abdomen, then the sacral region, and finally the cervix were subjected to the rays. The effects were both local and general. The catarrh of the cervix uteri healed, leukorrhœa first diminished and then ceased altogether, and the keratogenous action of the light produced a firm epithelium on the cervix. In this respect irradiation was more effective than lunar caustic treatment.

In cases of gonorrheal infection of the vagina irradiation, according to Heynemann, is beset with much difficulty on account of its inflammatory irritation. Wagner successfully treated gonorrhœa (and colpitis granularis), as did Liese, of Lübeck, who used irrigation in addition to irradiation. According to Wagner both the bactericidal properties of the rays and the effects of heat (by which the gonococci are destroyed) are instrumental in the treatment of gonorrhœa. After first cleansing the vagina and cervix with H_2O_2, the affected parts are irradiated for periods lasting from 1–6 minutes, at a distance of 5–6 inches (measuring from the edge of the inner hood aperture of the lamp to the entrance of the vagina), the surrounding area being carefully covered.

cf., Zentralblatt für Gynäkologie, No. 44, 1921.

F. M. Meyer* reports on the effect produced by X-rays and quartz light upon certain diseases of the sexual organs, and recommends, in conformity with the details given by Gauss, the use of general quartz light irradiations as an adjuvant to the customary treatment of gonorrhœa and non-specific discharge, which treatment proved successful. Another complaint which responds particularly to irradiation in contradistinction to all other therapeutic methods, is the soft phagedenic chancre. The disease is characterized by tendency to penetration, and is accompanied by an unpleasant odour and considerable pain. All treatment, including iodoform, gives at best only temporary improvement. The writer uses local quartz light irradiation in treating this disease, using the Kromayer Lamp for vaginal treatment in women. It is necessary to choose the shortest possible distance and to irradiate as long as possible, so that the bacteria are destroyed. Seeing that no other treatment cures the condition, the practitioner should not cease irradiations until complete cure has been brought about, which occurs in most instances. Naturally there are no objections to combining irradiation with other treatment.

In diseases of the vagina and the cervix the affected parts are made accessible by means of specula of wood, glass, or porcelain (not of metal), or else the ultra-violet light may be applied through quartz rods. The irradiation should be brief, *i.e.*, from 1–8 minutes only, to avoid irritating the sensitive mucous membranes. Erosions of the cervix, however, may be irradiated for longer periods (10–15 minutes), provided that the mucous membrane of the vagina is well protected by the speculum.

Diseases of the Uterus and Adnexa.

Wagner† recommends the artificial Alpine Sun quartz lamp for menstrual disorders, such as lumbago, menorrhagia, uterine myomas, and metrorrhagia caused thereby. He obtained good results by radiating the abdomen, the sacral region, and the cervix, using the aperture disc of the lamp and the speculum. Ostermann (Vienna) completely checked dysmenorrhœa by irradiation but could not accomplish much in cases of metrorrhagia. Fromme successfully used artificial Alpine Sun treatment for pyosalpinx. Thedering found that irradiation, especially the first

Zeitschrift für Urologie, No. 7 (1921).
†*Allgemeine Medizinische Zentralzeitung*, Nos. 5-6, 1913.

treatments, brought on the menses before they were quite due. He has treated such large numbers of women and young girls suffering from anæmia and its consequences (eczema, scrofula and tuberculosis), and has made this observation so frequently, that he has no longer any doubt as to the effects of general quartz light baths in promoting menstruation.

The contradiction between the observations of Wagner and Thedering is merely apparent. It is quite conceivable that irradiation of the abdominal organs increases the blood supply if there is a shortage of blood, yet have the opposite effect if there is an excess of it.

The writer has also obtained satisfactory results in cases of dysmenorrhea and pregnancy troubles (intumescence of the abdomen, stomach troubles, sickness). He was able to eliminate the last by cautious irradiation of the abdomen.

Landeker* conducted intravaginal and intrauterine irradiation with suitable applicators and reflecting devices for concentrating the rays in cases of congenital hypoplasia and hypo-function accompanied by oligomenorrhea or total amenorrhea, dysmenorrhea and infertility due to hypoplasia of the genitals or defective function of the ovaries, and also in climacterac neuroses of the sympathetic system and premature orgasm following operative or radiological castration ; using exposures of 10–20 minutes. In some characteristic cases of complete sexual coldness and disinclination for normal sexual relations, results in some few cases were permanent restoration to normal sexual feeling.

Apart from local irradiations of the vagina, the cervix, the external sexual organs, the abdomen, and the sacral region, general irradiations in the usual manner are also recommended for the treatment of abdominal diseases. They have proved especially helpful in cases complicated by simultaneous anæmia, tuberculosis, or scrofula. Further, they are of great assistance after operations, for assisting healing, and accelerating convalescence, and can be begun two or three days after the operation.

ECLAMPSIA.

Hochenbichler† recommends prophylactic treatment of eclampsia with the artificial Alpine Sun quartz lamp. Increase of blood

*Strahlentherapie, vol. xiv., 1922, No. 3.
†Monatsschr. f. Geburtshilfe u. Gynäkologie, vol. lxii.

pressure is amongst the most regular and certain symptoms of eclamptic predisposition, and for this reason measurements should always be made during pregnancy. Spasm of the renal vessels is reduced by quartz lamp irradiation, which increases the secretion of urine and diminishes albuminuria and the specific gravity of the urine. The earlier irradiation is administered, the better its effects. The treatment is also indicated immediately after birth, or in puerperal eclampsia ; general irradiations should be given twice daily, following the customary dosage.

MASTITIS.

Mastitis suppurativa is successfully treated by intensive irradiations at 12 inches distance of 5, 10, and 15 minutes' duration. Every case of incipient mastitis can be cured by suitable irradiation without abscess formation, according to Dr. Tauber.*

SUMMARY.

Established successes of artificial Alpine Sun treatment in Gynæcology :—

Wounds, granulations, ulcers, pruritus.

Vaginal catarrhs, cervix catarrhs, erosions of cervix, gonorrhœa.

Menstrual irregularities with and without hæmorrhage, uterine myomas, and metrorrhagia caused thereby.

Pregnancy troubles.

Post-operative for acceleration of healing and convalescence, especially if anæmia is present.

Results not fully established :—

Many kinds of gonorrhœa.

*Mediz. Klinik, May 8th, 1924.

Chapter VI

OPHTHALMOLOGY.

In the treatment of diseases of the eye with ultra-violet light opinions were at first divided, both as regards the nature and manner of the reaction of individual parts of the eye to the effects of light, and as regards the parts of the spectrum which were accountable for the changes observed. The injurious effects of light described as " ophthalmia electrica," the symptoms of which are acute photophobia, active lachrymation, conjunctivitis, dazzling sensations, lowered power of adaptation, and erythropsia after snow-blindness and diagnosed by Birch-Hirschfeld as central and para-central scotoma for green-red, from five patients; these, indeed, raise the question whether diseases of the eye were at all suitable for treatment by ultra-violet rays. These doubts were strengthened by the observation of Schanz, that the occurrence of cataract is to be ascribed to the action of ultra-violet rays. Only when it was established by the research work of various authorities that injury to the eye from ultra-violet radiation could be avoided by the use of suitable dosage, and that cataract was caused probably by the infra-red, and not by ultra-violet rays, was the subject of treatment of ocular diseases by ultra-violet radiation investigated more closely, when it was shown that various diseases of the eye could be successfully treated by this therapy.

There is no need here to go closely into the works of the authors who have discussed this question ; the names of Birch-Hirschfeld, Schanz, Jost, Vogt, Ogneff, Widmark, Hertel, Hess, Takamine, Takei, Hallauer, and others may be mentioned. Our purpose here is only to give some account of the therapeutic procedure, so far as it has proved suitable for use in this field.

Hitherto, with few exceptions, the objects of treatment have been the cornea and conjunctiva. When treating the conjunctiva, the eye-ball itself can be completely protected from the rays ; this is not the case when radiating the cornea. The latter procedure must therefore be carried out with special caution. The following diseases have up to now been successfully treated by irradiation :—

Serpiginous ulcer, eczematous and scrofulous conjunctivitis and keratitis, squamous and ulcerous blepharitis, hordeolum (sty), chalazion, lupus of the conjunctiva, trachoma marginal efflorescence, long-standing opacity of the cornea, tubercular and other infectious diseases of the eye.

The following publications call for notice :—

Strebel drew attention to the feasibility of treating gonorrheal processes with ultra-violet rays, and also of ameliorating inflammatory conditions of the eye by the production of local light-inflammation on the sclerotic or in close proximity to the eye.

Lundsgaard applied Finsen light in treating lupus of the conjunctiva. By means of special technique the lid is everted and pressed against the orbital margin with a pressure lens. The irradiations, which lasted from one to two hours, were in certain cases repeated up to ten times. The eye itself was protected by moist cotton wool. He has achieved good results, with only slight irritant effects.

Hertel used ultra-violet radiation from a cadmium-zinc arc for the treatment of serpiginous ulcer, and obtained satisfactory results. In comparing his technique with cauterization, he pointed out that the scars produced by his method were much finer. It was difficult to decide whether increased infiltrations were due to reaction after irradiation or to renewed activity of the disease.

Axmann treated a case of facial lupus, with severe chronic conjunctivitis and involvement of the cornea, by the Uviol Lamp, and observed reduction of the corneal opacity.

Hegner and Baumm in treating trachoma applied the radiation of the Kromayer Lamp by placing an applicator in direct contact with the palpebral conjunctiva. On the day following the first irradiation hyperæmia was observed, and on the second day a pseudo membrane formed. Stronger dosage resulted in œdema and swelling of the eyelid. Subsequently the membranes peeled off, and a smooth conjunctiva without any scar resulted. By this means, cures resulted in some cases.

Mohr and Baumm used an applicator similar in shape to a lid spatula, covering the side nearest the eye-ball with metal for protection. This treatment also resulted in the formation of a pseudo-membrane which disappeared again after a few days. They observed signs of reactive inflammation without pronounced necrosis. On the basis of their successful results, they recommend ultra-violet radiation for trachoma of very recent origin, and for obdurate follicular trachoma.

Schanz treated two cases of lupus with the quartz lamp, in front of which he placed a small trough of Uviol glass filled with Wood's solution.   He also irradiated infiltrations of the cornea, corneal ulcers, and pannus from lupus and trachoma.

Isaak irradiated cases of trachoma with the Finsen lamp and obtained satisfactory results.   Only in two cases of papillary trachoma with much infiltration and few follicles were the results less favourable.

Lundsgaard reported good results from Finsen light treatment of conjunctival tuberculosis ; in his experience, short sessions at infrequent intervals are sufficient.

Chotzen and Kunitzky irradiated the cornea by means of the quartz lamp and applicators in cases showing changes of trachomatous origin.   Prior to doing so, they had experimented on animals, and ascertained that apart from a reduction in the pigmentation of the iris no pathological change resulted.   They made these experiments with a large number of animals, subjecting them to clinical and pathological examination at intervals ranging from three hours to three weeks after the treatment.   In two cases of recent trachoma they obtained successful results, whereas an inveterate case showing extensive changes from the disease did not respond equally well.   A case of nodular keratitis, after showing temporary symptoms of irritation, also responded favourably to the treatment.   A case of progressive infiltration of the cornea promised well, but the treatment was abandoned before its completion.   Two cases of parenchymatous keratitis and one of irido-cyclitis remained unaffected, and in one case of scrofulous keratitis the effects were unfavourable.

More recently Passow has recommended irradiation with the artificial Alpine Sun quartz lamp for the treatment of persistent marginal efflorescence, ulcers, and infiltrations, and for reducing corneal opacities.   By experiments on animals he ascertained that the physical laws governing the chemical action of the rays also apply to their action on the eye.   Five minutes irradiation of a rabbit's eye at 24 inches distance injured neither the cornea nor the interior of the eye.   Therapeutic radiations of the same duration, at 32 inches distance, were effective without any harmful results.

Seefelder has achieved excellent results, using Passow's technique.

Pleikart Stumpf* confirms the data of Koeppe and Passow regarding the value of treatment with the artificial Alpine Sun quartz lamp in ophthalmology. He emphasizes the beneficial effect of ultra-violet therapy on photophobia, which frequently disappears after three or four irradiations. In his opinion, constitutional diseases of the eye should be treated by general rather than local irradiation.

Kraupa† used general irradiation with the artificial Alpine Sun in tuberculous diseases of the eye, with excellent results. He particularly observed the disappearance of other co-existent symptoms. Köllner, Filbrys, and Fischel‡ also report good results in these diseases by combined treatment with irradiation and partial antigen. Schnaudigel§ recommends, in addition to general irradiation, the administration of " Krysolgan."

Passow‖ and Birch-Hirschfeld¶ have reported on the treatment of infectious diseases of the eye.

According to Passow, in treating infectious eye diseases, primarily staphylococcal conditions, quartz light or iron arc light are preferable to carbon arc radiation on account of their richness in intense ultra-violet rays. The use of sensitizers is not necessary. As far as possible, the shorter ultra-violet rays, i.e., below 3000 A.U., should be used, as staphylococci manifest good powers of absorption for these particular rays.

Birch-Hirschfeld reports on the treatment by ultra-violet rays of infectious diseases of the cornea ; a number of other corneal affections have also responded well to irradiation. He has treated, by this means, 22 cases of diplo-bacillary ulcer, 48 cases of pannus ulcers, 30 cases of marginal ulcer, and 45 cases of particularly obdurate scrofulous ulcers ; and with few exceptions (the scrofulous cases showing least certain results), these were cured. The scars were characterized by special fineness. Superficial keratitis constitutes a further domain of irradiation therapy. In Birch-Hirschfeld's experience, abrasion followed the instilling of drops of fluorescin and application of irradiation brings strikingly good and speedy results.

*Archiv für Augenheilkunde, vol. xc., 1921, No. 1.
†Zeitschrift für Augenheilkunde, vol. xlii., 1919, No. 3.
‡Archiv für Augenheilkunde, vol. lxxxvii., 1920, Nos. 1-2.
§Münchener med. Wochenschrift, May 13th, 1921.
‖Archiv für Augenheilkunde, vol. xciii., 1923, Nos. 3-4.
¶Zeitschrift für Augenheilkunde, vol. liii.

Irradiation proved of special value also in recent, infected corneal injuries. The results were, however, less successful in keratitis, of the deep and tuberculous forms, and episcleritis. With interstitial keratitis, experiments with prolonged treatments, wider focus, increased intensity of radiation and screening-off of the shortest-waved rays, have yielded encouraging results. Birch-Hirschfeld comes to the conclusion that ultra-violet radiation has proved so valuable in the treatment of inflammatory corneal diseases that he now finds it indispensable. He increases the effect of irradiation by administration of drops of 2% solution of fluorescin. He usually irradiates twice daily, five to six minutes each, during about a fortnight, using carbon arc light focussed through a quartz lens. For the artificial Alpine Sun quartz lamp, the lamp distance would be from 32 to 40 inches.

Waubke, from whose report the above remarks are in large part taken, states the following as his conclusions reached from his work at Professor Stock's Eye Clinic :—

" Irradiation of the eye with ultra-violet has at this stage been used by comparatively few practitioners. Yet the beginnings made in this domain are so promising that further investigation will undoubtedly be made along the lines already opened, and many a question which is still obscure will certainly be cleared up.

" In practice, however, the quartz lamp will assuredly be used by all eye-clinics and many ophthalmologists for general therapeutic treatment ; particularly in eye diseases which have their origin in constitutional deficiency. In Professor Stock's Eye Clinic, we have for many years made the most extensive use of the Alpine Sun lamp. Following the technique which is fully stated in another section of this work, we have throughout given irradiation to all cases of scrofula ; all patients with endogenous tuberculosis of the eye ; cases of iritis, cyclitis, choroiditis ; children suffering from parenchymatous keratitis of syphilitic origin, so often in deplorable condition ; and, among other cases, those suffering from anæmia, malnutrition, and exhaustion ; in brief, all those cases which correspond to the indications stated in the general section of this work. Köppe reports in like terms of the work at the Halle Clinic. There, too, the scrofulous patients are the primary subjects of irradiation ; and in this regard it may be stated that Köppe has such children exposed to the lamp without goggles, but with their eyes closed, strict supervision being exercised in this regard. He has observed good effects on the eyelids, usually more or less involved in such cases, especially on acute inflammatory catarrh. The method is certainly unexceptionable, and the results good. With many of our patients, little or no treatment can be given to the eye itself, and just for this reason we must lay greatest stress on energetic general measures ; coupled with pharmaceutical and immunizing therapeutic measures, the Alpine Sun lamp is of value here through its action on appetite, metabolism, and sleep."

More recently, Professor Stock* has recommended irradiation with the artificial Alpine Sun lamp in treating scrofulous complaints.

Passow's Irradiation Technique.

Passow has in recent years further extended his technique, on which he reports in a notable paper.† He lays particular stress on the necessity of stating exact details as to the type of lamp, age of burner, line voltage, intensity of current, duration and lamp distance of each treatment, whenever results are published, to enable exact comparison.

He used an Alpine Sun quartz lamp at 110 volts (the amperage of the lamp is constant at the same voltage), applying general, local, and combined irradiation. The first were given every alternate day, at 24 inches distance, on both the front and back of the patient ; the first treatment being 5 minutes on each side, the second 10, and all subsequent sessions 15 minutes each. If no indications of general disease were present, he confined treatment to local irradiation at distances ranging from 24 to 40 inches according to the sensitivity of the eye. The first session lasted 5 minutes ; and later sessions were determined from the degree of reaction experienced, with a maximum of 10 minutes. The lids were everted and a hand diaphragm used to ensure that only the diseased area, not the whole orbit, was exposed to the rays. Both methods were sometimes combined.

Passow's chief subject was scrofula, and the results obtained in treating over 100 children were uniformly good. In about a third

*Klinische Monatsblätter für Augenheilkunde, vol. lxxvi., 1926.
†Strahlentherapie, vol. xii., 1921.

of the total number, improvement was noticeable after the first, in the majority of the remainder after the second or third treatment, whilst in a few instances it did not set in till later. Irradiation was almost the only therapy used throughout, which fact is naturally important in estimating the value of the results. In diseases of the inner eye, primarily tuberculosis, he was unable to establish any definite results.

CHAPTER VII.

DISEASES OF THE EAR, THROAT AND NOSE.

According to Cemach,* of Vienna, "quartz light treatment appears destined to give effective assistance to the established methods in otology, and in some cases to supplant them where they have proved inadequate." He uses quartz light for treatment of the drum and middle ear, his method being that round quartz pencils of 5 mm. diameter, slightly rounded at the end, are adapted to the quartz window of the Kromayer Lamp and introduced into the external auditory meatus. For the treatment of operation cavities quartz rods of various diameters are used. In order most suitably to introduce the rods and to avoid injuries to the passage, the Kromayer lamp is attached to a rotatable stand so that the rod can be accurately centred before insertion into the canal. Short exposures, increased gradually, weak intensities of radiation, and the use of filters are recommended in order to avoid painful reactions in the ear.

For treating the larynx, Cemach has now gone over to direct irradiation with quartz light, having had unsatisfactory results from using Heusner's quartz applicators or Ladebeck and Noll's quartz mirrors for introducing ultra-violet rays. His results were thoroughly satisfactory ; infiltrations were reduced, ulcers healed up and scarred. Severe and extensive morbid processes were almost or entirely resolved. The effect on dysphagia was excellent, even in terminal cases. In the main, he treated tubercular conditions, and used at the same time suitable diet, hygienic measures, the rest cure (to a limited extent), and specific means (*i.e.*, tuberculomucin prepared by Weleminsky's method). But even without the aid of specific therapy he cured laryngeal tuberculosis by quartz light irradiation alone.†

*" Das Quarzlicht im Dienste der Ohrenheilkunde," *Klinischtherapeut. Wochenschrift,* vol. xxvi., No. 45/46.

†*Zeitschrift f. Hals-, Nasen- u. Ohrenheilk.,* vol. x., 1924.

For direct laryngeal irradiation with quartz light he uses the Photostat* to the Kromayer lamp designed by himself, shown in Fig. 23. This Photostat obviates all the defects which rendered irradiation of the larynx difficult and uncertain, so that by its aid even protracted laryngeal treatments can be carried out with full assurance and without undue inconvenience to the patient. Pressure on the teeth is avoided by setting the axis of the

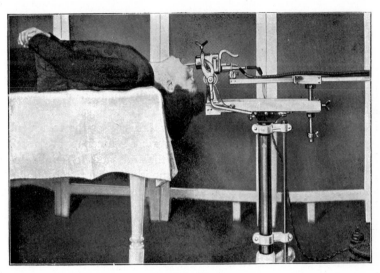

FIG. 23.

The Cemach Photostat in use.

speculum tube on the heavy stand, so that the teeth are not required to carry any weight, and the patient can easily shift pressure, should it occur, by slightly stretching the head. The Kromayer lamp is attached to the same stand in such a way that it is self-adjusting to the correct alignment relative to the larynx and sends its rays straight down it. By means of the Photostat, phototherapy of laryngeal diseases is freed of all difficulties for the practitioner.†

*Photostat is manufactured by Messrs. Reiner, of Vienna, whilst the quartz applicators, holders, etc., like the Kromayer Lamp itself, are Hanau-Hanovia products.

†Zur Technik der Quarzlichttherapie der Kehlkopftuberkulose. *Folia Otolaryngologica*, 1925.

The apparatus is also suitable for purposes of laryngeal exploration or operation, and affords a complete substitute for every other means of direct laryngoscopy. The larynx tube and its appropriate adjustment can be removed from the field of radiation by a handle, whereby the apparatus can be used for treating skin diseases and other external morbid processes. When the Cemach holder is affixed to the lamp, and the proper spring mounted applicator inserted, this serves for irradiation of the nose, the ear, mouth and tonsils, as well as for treatment of the eye, the urethra (using the special urethral applicator), and by means of special vaginal applicators or speculum tubes it can be used in gynæcological work.

Cemach begins with 1–2 minutes and gives treatments three times weekly, increasing by 1–2 minutes each time up to a dose of 10 minutes. This is as a rule sufficient. With patients who tolerate the treatment well he prefers to conclude with an irradiation of filtered (*i.e.*, blue) light, which is both less irritating and more penetrating. For this purpose the lamp is somewhat withdrawn and the blue filter inserted. The duration of this blue ray treatment depends on that of the white : *e.g.*, 5 minutes white, 5 minutes blue, making 10 minutes in all ; but may last longer. In general, he has seldom exceeded 20 minutes altogether. In cases of dysphagia, only blue light is used.

Powerful reaction is no drawback, yet his endeavour is to avoid this, in order not to upset the patient's general condition by an onset of pain. When the procedure outlined above is adhered to, strong reactions seldom occur. Should an overdose take place, treatment must be discontinued until all pain has subsided.

Regarding the capacities of the Photostat, in phototherapy of laryngeal tuberculosis, Cemach expresses the opinion* that the best therapy for this disease is a combination of the most effective local curative treatment, *i.e.*, direct irradiation, with systematic general treatment. For direct irradiation, the means comprise ultra-violet light, which has a stimulant-irritant action, whilst the filtered blue light serves to tone down the effects of the ultra-violet. In acute cases, this therapy may be assisted by the use of the Sollux Lamp. The general treatment must be suited to

*Address to the Sixth Session of the Gesellschaft Deutscher Hals-, Nasen- und Ohrenärzte, Hamburg, May 20th, 1926.

the circumstances of the special case ; in exudative pulmonary conditions protective measures, such as rest, open air, and change of climate ; in cirrhotic processes stimulation therapy of every description (tuberculin, sunlight, artificial light baths), and exercise, should be employed, and varied according to the stages of the pulmonary and laryngeal conditions as necessary.

In tuberculosis of the middle ear, which is an osseous tuberculosis like any other, Cemach obtained good results from general light baths and artificial Alpine Sun treatment ; also in scrofulous diseases, particularly scrofulous eczema. In perichondritis, the prognosis is very much improved when quartz light is used. By combined irradiation with Sollux and quartz lamps, Cemach was able to cure such cases in two to four weeks with good cosmetic results, the cartilage being preserved. Successes are especially marked in incipient or developing cases of perichondritis.

Traumatic lesions of the lobe of the ear caused by cuts or shots, as well as necrotic processes after frostbite, burns, or chemical action, heal much more rapidly and with better cosmetic results under irradiation than similar cases treated by other means.

A case of tuberculosis cutis of the lobe of the ear healed within three months under quartz light, without leaving the slightest malformation.

In cases of otitis externa quartz light irradiation eases the pain, checks inflammation, and promotes resorption, with better results than those attainable by established methods. The Sollux lamp, with its luminous heat rays, is more advantageous here than the quartz lamp.

Imhofer successfully irradiated cases of otitis in babies with the artificial Alpine Sun.* He uses it in those instances where the disease is torpid from the outset, or becomes torpid at an early stage, where the secretion assumes a mucopurulent character, or remains so in unchanged amount, without displaying marked reactive symptoms. In such cases he achieved rapid diminution of the secretion by quartz light, provided that the case was not one of caries. He further mentions the successful results of Sollux lamp irradiation in this condition, on which Gerstenberger and Dodge have also written.

*Med. Klinik, No. 26, 1925.

Eczema of the auditory meatus, like other forms, and chronic ulcerous myringitis, are quickly and permanently cured by means of quartz light.

Treatment of middle ear processes by quartz light is restricted in scope, on account of inaccessibility, although even in these conditions it is not without effect. Cemach therefore endeavoured to obtain indirect effects by means of long-waved rays (carbon arc light and Sollux lamp radiation).

In a more recent report* Cemach expressed the view that helio-therapy, *i.e.*, sunlight, quartz light, and carbon arc radiation, is capable of curing aural tuberculosis " of any type, at any stage, and at any age."

In acute otitis media simplex, and acute exudative catarrh of the middle ear, quartz light treatment supplants the usual anti-phlogistic measures. Luminous heat, as from the Sollux lamp, is particularly favourable in its analgesic action. Paracentesis is seldom necessary in cases of otitis media when irradiation is used.

In acute mastoiditis, early mastoid process symptoms can often be subdued by intensive irradiation without the necessity of operation.

Views are divided concerning the success of quartz light treatment in chronic suppuration of the middle ear ; splendid results on the one hand being balanced by complete failures on the other.

Favourable results follow the application of quartz light to the chronic adhesive processes in the tympanic cavity, which are the cause of permanent functional disturbances. In these conditions the softening action of the rays on scars develops its effect in loosening and resolving the adhesions. Cemach succeeded in improving patients' hearing from six to eight times, but only in cases where the adhesions occurred at a spot accessible to the irradiation.

Kragh, of the Finsen Institute, Copenhagen, achieved strikingly good results in seven out of fifteen cases of otosclerosis by means of quartz light, although only after treatment had been continued for eighteen months or even longer.

Special mention should be made of the tonic action of general quartz light baths on patients exhausted and debilitated from

*Wiener medizinische Wochenschrift, No. 7, 1921.

intracranial complications, especially from protracted sepsis. The excellent action of light on metabolism, circulation, appetite and nutrition are well seen here.

Scheffer* cured four out of five cases of purulent otitis media in tuberculous patients with the artificial Alpine Sun quartz lamp. In five other cases where suppuration had persisted for twenty years, this itself was unaffected, but the evil odour disappeared.

Dosage : Commence with 10 minutes at 10 inches distance ; even at the third and fourth treatments prolong exposure to three-quarters of an hour, diminishing the distance to 6 or 4 inches.

Technique : A funnel of celluloid (not metal, as this might become too hot) is inserted deeply into the ear, adjusted to the ear drum and the perforation. The face and throat are covered, and the outer ear smeared with some protective ointment to which a little aqueous solution of acid vaseline has been added.

Lautenschläger and Adler† have experimentally investigated the action of ultra-violet rays and their therapeutic uses in laryngology, using various ultra-violet sources (the acetylene lamp, the quartz lamp, electric filament lamps and unenclosed electric carbon filaments). Their conclusion is that although it may be possible to obtain disinfectant action from irradiation, provided this is sufficiently protracted, the practical applicability of this is very restricted as regards the mouth cavity, since sterilization to the extent of destruction of germs located in the fissures of the tonsils appears impossible. Further, ultra-violet rays appear to have an anæsthetic effect ; at any rate, they can produce areflexia in the sense of Spiess' theory of inflammation.

From a summary of literature kindly lent by Dr. Koch, of the University Ear Clinic, Erlangen, it is evident that local application of the artificial Alpine Sun in diseases of the throat and ear is scanty up to now, and mainly restricted to suppurative processes which can be made accessible to ultra-violet rays.

It may also be mentioned here that Professor E. Friedberger and Dr. E. Shioji‡ have recommended direct irradiation of the mouth cavity in bacterial infections. In experiments on rabbits,

---

Beiträge zur Klinik der Tuberkulose, Eighth Supplement.

† (*Archiv für Laryngologie,* vol. xxix. 1915).

‡*Deutsche med. Wochenschrift,* 1914, No. 12.

they observed very active destruction of bacteria through direct introduction of ultra-violet rays immediately into the cavity.

Blust employed ultra-violet rays for disinfection of the mouth cavity in gingivitis and pyorrhœa. His opinion is that with the combination of dental surgery and ultra-violet treatment, a most important part is played by light owing to its action in increasing blood supply through the hyperæmia and invigorating the activity and metabolism of the tissues.

Ladebeck has described* a laryngeal quartz mirror, which can be used by the patient himself for sunlight irradiation of diseases of the larynx, and by the doctor for irradiation of other areas, e.g., the pharynx, by due use of the head band lamp with a quartz mirror, which does not absorb the ultra-violet rays.

Dosage with the artificial Alpine Sun should, when used for irradiation in the mouth, be weak at the outset and increased with caution.

In diseases of the ear and throat, since it is often a question of tuberculosis or scrofula, general irradiation with the artificial Alpine Sun should be administered in addition to local, in order to improve the patient's general condition through the general action of quartz light and thus assist the cure of the local process. The general irradiation should be administered according to the dosage stated in Part I.

It may again be mentioned that treatment with quartz rods is only possible with the Kromayer lamp.

Dr. J. L. Kyers† reports on the treatment of hay fever with quartz light. He uses the Kromayer lamp with a quartz rod for endonasal treatment, giving doses of 2–10–12 minutes, combined with general irradiation with the Alpine Sun. In his view, the local irradiation is greatly assisted by the general light bath. From two years' experience, this procedure, although not entirely specific for hay fever, has shown a high percentage of cures, and more can be achieved thereby than by any other therapeutic method.

As indications for endonasal quartz light therapy, Dr. Cemach‡ holds that only the following can be accepted at present : hay

---

*Münch. med. Wochenschrift, 1920, No. 50.

†" The Quartz Lamp."

‡Monatsschr. f. Ohrenheilk. u. Laryngo-Rhinologie, No. 4, 1925.

fever, ozæna, and nasal tuberculosis. In treating hay fever and ozæna, he uses the following procedure and technique* :—

The apparatus, externally resembling the Photostat, consists essentially of two portions : a transmission device which conducts the rays into the interior of the nose ; and mechanism by which precise adjustment of the lamp and the attached device to the desired spot is made possible.

As a means of transmission, after many experiments a quartz rod flattened on both sides has proved most suitable, as it conducts the rays with minimum loss of intensity. Systematic endonasal quartz light therapy was, however, only made possible when Cemach devised a loose connection of the applicator to the lamp. The introduction of a rigid quartz rod into the nose was in many cases prevented by irregularities of the septum or prominent muscles ; only when the nose is wide, as in ozæna, can a rigid applicator be employed. The spring-mounted rod, guided by the hand of the operator, can be introduced, and with practice can be taken to the back of the pharynx without the slightest inconvenience to the patient, unless some exceptional malformation of the septum is present.

A special holder serves for attachment of the spring-mounted applicator to the Kromayer lamp, and incorporates a device for filtration of the rays.

The mechanism consists of a stand with rack and pinion fittings, which facilitate regular and easy adjustment of the lamp both horizontally and vertically. This form of stand was devised by Dr. Cemach some years ago for irradiation of the ear. The new " Photostat " apparatus, constructed to the design of Dr. Cemach for laryngeal treatment, is also suitable for nasal therapy.

Endonasal irradiation is conducted as follows : The nasal membrane is desensitized with 20% cocaine solution, to which adrenalin may be added when treating ozæna, but not on any account for hay fever. The nose is carefully cleansed from mucus and crusts ; the crusts of ozæna must in particular be removed from the fissures and central nasal passage. Caution is necessary here ; the membrane must not be made to bleed, as blood absorbs the ultra-violet rays.†

*Address to the Vienna Laryngo-rhinologische Gesellschaft on March 3rd, 1925.

†The best means of removing crusts is by levering them up with a probe, made with a thick head.

The applicator itself must be scrupulously cleaned with a pad of moist cotton wool when repeatedly used, special care being taken that no particles of mucus are left adhering to the flat surfaces.*

The tip of the nose, upper lip, and adjacent areas, which are exposed to the lateral radiation from the conical portion of the rod, are best shielded by means of a protective ointment, such as " Protectol." Care must be taken that the applicator does not become smeared. When blue light is used, ointment is not necessary.

For fixation of the head, some support is required, fastened to a heavy chair ; it should be such as to allow of different positions, including full extension of the neck.

When the nose is wide, as in ozæna, the rod can be introduced in any position of the head. When the lumen is narrow, and particularly when irregularly shaped, the passage must first be determined by rhinoscopy, the ascertained direction projected on to the surface of the skull, and the head then so placed that this line lies in a horizontal plane.

After the patient's head has been so fixed, the apparatus is brought up and so placed that the quartz rod is pointing directly at one nostril. The operator stands at the left side of the stand, his right hand governing the rack and pinion mechanism, whilst his left grasps the applicator holder from the front in such a manner that the rod lies along the half-extended index finger. The lamp is now racked horizontally forward until the rod touches the upper lip, and then raised by means of the other cogwheel as far as is allowed by the tip of the nose, the resistance of which is overcome by the help of the index finger assisting. With this, the tip of the applicator enters the vestibule, and need only be racked forward to penetrate into the nasal cavity, during which operation the forefinger is used to help it past the upward protuberance of the limen nasi. This stage is facilitated if the vestibule is illuminated with mild blue light from the applicator so that the operation is done under visual control. Further obstacles are overcome in the same way with the help of the finger, which can explore the nasal passage by very slight pendulatory movements and find a clear way. The whole procedure hardly occupies ten seconds.

*The rod can be boiled, but the spring suffers if boiled repeatedly. It is therefore advisable to use separate applicators for ozæna and hay fever, which can be distinguished by etching the letters O and H on the inner surfaces ; cleansing with water and alcohol is then sufficient.

The shutter is now fully opened, the filter being interposed if necessary, and irradiation commenced. During its course, the applicator is gradually withdrawn, the rate of withdrawal being suited to the period of irradiation. To take an example : With an exposure of five minutes the end of the rod, which is 5 cm. long, is withdrawn about 1 cm. per minute ; a centimetre scale is etched on the upper side.

After irradiation, the nose is greased. Nasal plugs of ointment are best, to be left in place for one to two hours, made to the formula :—

Rp.	Alum. acet. bas. soluti	...	...	5.0
	Adip. lanæ anhydr.	...	...	...	10.0
	Vasel. amer. albi	...	...	...	20.0
	Ol. rosae gtt. II.	...	...	...	M.f.u.*

The technique is very different for hay fever and ozæna.

In hay fever treatment the basic principle is not to irritate. No reaction must be set up, as this will intensify the inflammatory symptoms instead of diminishing them. On the other hand, irradiation must not be too weak, or no results will be obtained. The optimum dose corresponds roughly to the least perceptible stimulation ; this, however, varies to an extraordinary extent. In general, the membrane in cases of hay fever is oversensitive, and minimal amounts of irradiation will achieve the object. Some cases, on the other hand, require doses many times greater ; the experienced practitioner will discover these after the first treatment.

Cemach, in treating hay fever, uses exclusively blue light ; *i.e.*, filtered quartz light, in which the shortest, chemical and highly irritant ultra-violet rays are lacking, and which therefore is much milder in its effects. A small Uviol filter is incorporated in the applicator holder, and is switched in by means of a lever.

An exact dosage cannot be given, as lamps do not operate at the same intensity, a new Kromayer lamp being two to three

*The following is a good way of introducing the ointment stopping into the nose : A small bar of metal, size $120 \times 10 \times 1$ mm., well polished and nickelled, and rounded off at the front end, is wound evenly with cotton wool over the front half, the end of the wool being caught up in winding. This is charged with ointment and inserted into the nose ; then press the nostrils to retain the wool and withdraw the bar. To be left in position for an hour.

times more powerful than one which has been long in use. Dosage is here given according to light-minutes.

If a new lamp is used, begin with $1\frac{1}{2}$, or at most 2 minutes, in each nostril. If no reaction follows, give twice the dose two days later. If a weak reaction occurs (slight increase of secretion, and slight burning setting in four to five hours after the irradiation) and if improvement follows next day, however slight (*e.g.*, diminished conjunctival irritation), then the next dose, given two to three days after the first, is made a minute longer, and subsequent doses increased by the same amount and given at equal intervals ; a more rapid increase is sometimes possible. If strong reaction occurs (acute rhinitis) it is most advisable to wait until it has completely subsided and then test cautiously for the point of minimum stimulation. In many cases the correct dose is then found to be the same.

Every practitioner must work according to his experience of his own lamp, and perhaps according to the local character of the disease, and treat each case on individual lines. The chief thing is to bear in mind the principle that procedure must be conservative and gradual, and dosage cautious although not too timid.

With ozæna, the procedure is diametrically opposite. This severe condition can only be influenced by large amounts of pure quartz light, and the caustic action of the short-waved rays appears to be decisive. The ozæna membrane is often strikingly insensitive even to the shortest ultra-violet rays, and in many cases Cemach could not reach the point of reaction under 15 minutes.

Technique accordingly consists in intense irradiation with white light (unfiltered quartz light). Treatment must be followed by a reaction. The stronger the reaction, the better the result. The limit will be determined by the individual sensitivity, and it is not necessary to cause undue pain ; care is particularly advisable in the ethmoidal region, as a certain amount of undue reaction in this area may easily cause headaches. On the other portions of the nasal membrane even severe reactions are harmless, as they do no more than cause burns and the sensation of heat which can be allayed by the application of grease does not inconvenience even delicate patients.

Whilst, when treating hay fever, a single radiation of each nostril with the head held upright is often sufficient, and the entire session lasts only a few minutes, with ozæna each side must be treated several times, so that the irradiation, with preparation and after-treatment, requires on the average half-an-hour. The intense caustic action of the quartz light is only effective on the places which are exposed directly to the rays. Diffuse irradiations are therefore insufficient ; the lower and upper parts of the nose must be treated in different positions. After three to five sessions the nose is fairly well deodorised, and at this stage the practitioner can find by investigation of the crusts at which spots fœtor is still present. Special attention is then given to these areas. As a rule the middle of the nasal duct or fissures prove refractory, as it is difficult to make the light penetrate here. Ways and means must be found to radiate these areas also ; *e.g.*, by bending the head back to the fullest possible extent, turning the head sideways, and so forth. All things considered, the treatment of ozæna is long and wearisome, and requires not only experience, but also watchfulness and patience.

Here again it is impossible to state exact rules for dosage. The following may be taken as guiding lines : Start with 2 minutes each on the lower and upper parts, and increase at each session by 2 minutes below and 1 minute above until strong reaction occurs. After treatment, and on the day following, apply a plug of ointment. The next session after the reaction has subsided, three to six days later.

The number of sessions necessary varies greatly. As an average, experience has taught the writer to reckon on about ten ; when the condition is of medium severity, this number has always been sufficient.

When to stop treatment is a matter of experience ; it is hard to define a standard time. The appearance of the membrane and secretion, the formation of crusts, the patient's own feelings, and so forth, must be considered together. In mild cases where atrophy is not great the question is easy, as soon as no further crust formation is perceptible ; it is, however, certainly advisable to give a few further doses of radiation at longer intervals even after all symptoms of disease have disappeared. In doubtful cases a short observation period should intervene, and if necessary treatment should be resumed without undue loss of time. Observation for several months is recommended in all cases.

Cemach characterizes the action of radiation, in relation to the three cardinal symptoms, as follows :—

1. Fœtor was permanently eradicated in 18 cases, and in the remaining 7 cases disappeared for a time. Even in cases where crust formation persisted (see below), no perceptible odour remained; the crusts which may form are either entirely odourless, or have a slightly rancid smell where inadequate care has been taken, but in no instance could the characteristic ozæna smell be detected.

2. The atrophy is not affected by radiation treatment. In a few cases where little atrophy had occurred, in which both the fœtor and the crust-formation disappeared entirely, Cemach believes he has ascertained a consecutive increase of volume of the membrane a long time after cessation of treatment. In one case the diminution in size of the cavity was particularly striking, and the atrophy could hardly be detected a year after treatment. In the overwhelming majority of cases, however, this regeneration does not take place.

3. Crust formation is affected in different ways; in general, it is dependent on the grade of atrophy.

(a) A majority of cases with little atrophy (6 out of 8) remained free of crusts. They had to continue douching for some time (two to three months), but were then able gradually to discontinue this without a recurrence. The two oldest cases of this description have remained free of crusts for 19 and 13 months respectively without douching. All six patients remained free of inconvenience from the disease, and considered themselves cured. Two cases, on the other hand, were still obliged to douche the nose from time to time $5\frac{1}{2}$ and 8 months after treatment had stopped, as otherwise slight formation of crusts occurred.

(b) A majority of cases with atrophy of medium degree (4 out of 6) are still subject to slight crust-formation. The four patients could, however, obviate this by daily douching with a solution of common salt or soda. With the other two a crust occurs now and then, which disappears spontaneously and is free of smell.

(c) Where atrophy is of advanced degree (4 cases), crust formation continues, but to a smaller extent than before irradiation and as a rule irregularly. The nose often remains almost or quite free of crusts for weeks together, and then from some cause (*e.g.*, a chill) these recur in large amount. Daily douching does not avail to prevent their formation. As a rule a large composite crust is discharged in 8–10 days, which is, however, always odourless or only slightly rancid.

In summary, the action of irradiation is as follows :—

The chief symptom of ozæna, which gives the disease its special stamp and constitutes the main trouble of the subject, the fœtor, can be effectively dealt with by the endonasal application of quartz light. The symptoms of atrophic rhinitis, however, withstand this treatment ; the atrophy cannot be affected, and the formation of crusts only when atrophy is of slight degree. In other words : With ozæna in the initial stages, or of long subsistence but accompanied by only a mild degree of atrophy, clinical results which are completely satisfactory can be obtained. In advanced cases pronounced improvement of the condition is feasible.

Sollux Lamp Irradiation.

For light treatment in otology the luminous heat rays of the Sollux lamp are used with success, as mentioned above, in addition to quartz light. Oeken* reports as under on this subject, from observation of 258 cases :—

The patient being seated in an easy basket chair, the Sollux lamp, which is universally adjustable, is directed on the ear from a distance of 4 inches, and radiation given for a period averaging one hour. The eyes are protected by goggles which are free of metal parts. The Sollux lamp effect consists in a deep penetrating hyperæmia of the ear and its neighbourhood, which is of long duration. Oeken knows of no contra-indications.

In acute otitis media simplex Oeken achieved the following results with four to six treatments : pain was immediately relieved, paracentesis was avoided, and duration of cure was shortened, on a conservative estimate, by at least one-third.

In acute perforative otitis media the ear was radiated daily after being cleansed. From the fifth day on an air douche is used and hydrogen peroxide dropped in, this being then mopped with wool and a wool stopping inserted. After an average of ten treatments several advantages follow : the pains vanish after the first

---

* " Anwendung der Wärmestrahlen in der Ohrenheilkunde," *Therap. Halbmonstshefte*, 1, xii., 1920, No. 23.

radiation ; the course of the disease is easier and shorter, and the ear drum heals in every case with scarcely a visible scar. Every case which was complicated by acute mastoiditis was cured through daily radiation. Two cases of simple incision were cured in 16 days through radiation with very little scar formation.

In acute exudative catarrh of the middle ear, also, irradiation has shown good results. The following advantages attach to this method : (1) paracentesis is avoided ; (2) the duration of treatment is reduced to half in comparison with former methods, and the disease is prevented from passing into chronic catarrh of the middle ear ; and (3) the capacity of hearing is fully restored.

In a case of hæmatoma auris, the tumour was reduced by half after five treatments, and disappeared entirely after ten. The other treatment used consisted in protective bandaging.

In otitis externa circumscripta irradiation showed the following results : (1) all cases were freed of pain after the first treatment ; (2) a third of the cases were healed without suppuration intervening ; (3) the number of radiations varied from two to six ; (4) in no case was incision necessary, as softening set in early and the plug of pus could be expelled by slight pressure ; (5) the duration of cure was shortened in all cases, and relapses were avoided.

Lithiasis of the submaxillary gland was cured by Cemach with 14 Sollux radiations, after extrusion of the calculus.*

SUMMARY.

Proved successes from quartz light irradiation in diseases of the throat and ear.

(From local irradiation).

Dermatoses (scrofulous eczema), alopecia, wounds, ulcers, abscesses, local gangrene (especially after frostbite), keloid, tuberculosis of the middle ear, tuberculosis cutis of the outer ear, otitis externa, chronic ulcerative myringitis, simple acute inflammation of the middle ear, acute mastoiditis ; chronic adhesive processes in the tympanic cavity. Gingivitis ; pyorrhœa.

Successes not fully established :

Chronic suppuration of the middle ear, and diseases of the mouth cavity.

*Monatsschr. f. Ohrenheilkunde, No. 12, 1924.

For irradiation in the auditory canal quartz rods are used, or the area to be treated is made accessible to the rays by means of a celluloid funnel.

———

In addition to local irradiation, general light baths improve the patient's general condition and assist the cure of the local process.

Established successes from luminous heat irradiation with the Sollux Lamp.

Acute simple otitis media, acute perforative inflammation of the middle ear, acute mastoiditis, acute exudative catarrh of the middle ear, hæmatoma auris, otitis externa circumscripta, lithiasis of the submaxillary gland.

CHAPTER VIII.

DENTAL SURGERY.

ACCORDING to Professor Seidel,* of Marburg, the artificial Alpine Sun, or rather quartz light, may be used in dental surgery :—

1. For " bleaching " teeth.
2. For treating inflammatory and suppurative conditions in the oral cavity.
3. For softening scars in the mouth.

By means of quartz rods, which are pressed firmly against the membrane, penetrating treatment can be given with the rays, and the area treated can be determined from the shape of the rod. These rods can be fastened quite simply by means of screws immediately in front of the window of the Kromayer lamp. A long rod ground from crystal quartz free from bubbles, bent, conical or straight as may be, is sufficient. The conical applicator is 100 mm. long, with a diameter of 29·34 mm. at the base and tapering to 12·15 at the tip, which is flat, but rounded off at the edges. The rays are to some extent concentrated through the conical shape, so that nearly all rays which enter the thick base emerge from the smaller tip. The rod serves both for softening scars and for bleaching teeth. The straight rod is also 100 mm. long, by 12 mm. thick, and serves for the same purposes, particularly when the mouth is small, while the curved rod is for regions otherwise difficult of access.

A quartz rod intended for dental surgery should satisfy the following requirements :—

1. It should lose as little light as possible between the lamp window and the treatment end.
2. The amount of light sent out at the treatment end should be as great as possible, as the duration of a treatment which postulates holding the mouth open continuously is restricted.

*" Zahnärztliche Lichttherapie mit Quecksilberbogenlampen und Quarzstäben," *Deutsche Zahnheilkunde, Forschung und Praxis,* 1920.

3. Its shape should be suitable for as wide a range of application as possible.

4. In order to be useful for " bleaching," the rod must give as even as possible a field of radiation at some distance from the treatment end, which field should not be much greater than the end itself ; the rays must therefore emerge parallel or nearly so.

5. The rod must allow of the compression treatment of the membrane.

6. It must be so shaped as not to be too brittle.

THERAPEUTIC APPLICATION.

Although this does not come directly under the heading of dental surgery, mention may here be made of irradiation with the artificial Alpine Sun in suppurative, ichorous, and malodorous injuries to the face and jaw, by which treatment the foul smell is soon lost and epithelial formation proceeds rapidly. Irradiation is administered, under the ordinary precautions (protection of the eyes), daily or every alternate day, lasting 5 to 10 minutes at 50 to 60 cm. distance.

1. Treatment of inflammatory and suppurative conditions. In addition to the biological action of ultra-violet rays, their bactericidal effect is here utilized. Disinfection of the oral cavity, or success in treating pyorrhœa alveolaris, cannot, however, be achieved by their use. Only the treatment of inflammatory and suppurative local conditions in the oral cavity promises success, and is carried out in the same way as the irradiation of every other kind of wound.

2. Treatment of scars in the mouth. Here we have to deal with those old, ropy scars extending over the cheeks, which obstruct opening of the mouth and often set up grave disturbances, and which defeat all extension measures and other surgical treatment.
Only the Kromayer lamp can be used. In order to obtain penetrative action and prevent irritation of the membrane, the blue filter must always be interposed. If possible, the thick conical applicator should be used, which sends the largest quantity of radiation into the tissues in the shortest time. Only if this cannot

be introduced on account of its thickness, should recourse be had to the straight or curved rods. The patient is directed to keep the scar strongly pressed against the applicator. The firmer the pressure, the better the deep action. The lamp is used fastened to its stand, the patient's head being to some extent jammed between the head-rest and the lamp.

The first radiation must not last longer than three minutes. At intervals of 2–3 days, treatment is prolonged by increases of 2–3 minutes up to 20 minutes. The 20 minutes treatment is then continued for some weeks. If irradiation has to be interrupted from any cause for longer than three or four days, a new start must be made with a short exposure. After a few weeks it is already seen that the tissues which were hard and empty of blood, are again soft and red. It is good at the same time to give stretching treatment with one of the well-known apparatus.

The entire course of treatment lasts about two months in severe cases. Relapses have not been observed ; on the contrary, there is always a powerful and beneficial after-action.

Only the Kromayer lamp is suitable for use with quartz applicators.

According to Leix,* ultra-violet rays are chiefly used in dental surgery for after-treatment following surgical procedure, and for bleaching discoloured teeth. Irradiation should be conducted immediately after the operation, in connection with cystectomy, osteotomy, incisions of the membranes, etc. In pyorrhœa alveolaris great improvement is obtained by opening up the membrane and destroying the granulation tissue. Irritation of the dental pulp is also successfully irradiated without removal of root fillings ; and the same is true of periodontitis, after the gangrenous matter has been removed from the canal ; of diseases of the maxillary fissure arising from dental causes ; trismus due to difficult dentition ; and softening of scars after maxillary resection. Ultra-violet radiation possesses, in short, pronounced curative action in all inflammatory diseases of the oral cavity, and affords alleviation of pain to the patient.

According to Leix, only such teeth can be bleached as have been discoloured by organic substances. If discoloration is due to metals or metallic salts, any attempt at bleaching is hopeless.

*Fortschrift d. Zahnheilk., vol. i., 1925.

For this treatment, the root filling must be made absolutely tight, and the cavity thoroughly cleaned and disinfected ; the application of an elastic stretcher is advisable. Using the Kromayer lamp, the surgeon irradiates for not more than 1½ minutes, increased later up to 5 minutes, quartz applicators being used to direct the light immediately upon the area to be treated.

Advanced degrees of stomatitis with gangrenous destruction of the gingiva were also cured by Leix through irradiation with the Kromayer lamp. Irradiation was given until reddening of the gums occurred ; *i.e.*, a stimulation dose, after preliminary treatment with hydrogen peroxide and alcohol.

SUMMARY.

Established successes of quartz light treatment in dental surgery.

For " bleaching " the teeth.

For treatment of inflammatory and suppurative diseases of the oral cavity.

For softening scars in the oral cavity.

In dental surgery, quartz applicators are essential.

––––––––––

Good results have also been obtained in dental surgery with luminous heat ray treatment from the Hanovia Sollux lamp, as in diseases of the ear and throat. The action of Sollux irradiation, as mentioned before, consists in the production of powerful hyperæmia, of deep penetration and long duration. The irradiated area and its surroundings are intensely reddened and suffused with blood. (Dr. Oeken.) The lamp is so directed upon the diseased area that the diseased focus lies at the centre of the field of light. Unfiltered light (without the coloured filter) produces hyperæmia ; blue light, when the blue filter is interposed, anæmia. The distance of the skin from the cork ring should be as short as the patient can possibly stand without undue inconvenience from the radiated heat ; *i.e.*, about six inches at the first treatment, and later five to three.

When the conical reflector extension is used with the large Sollux lamp it is essential to switch in about one-third of the series resistance. When the small Cemach Sollux lamp is in use, the lamp must never be covered by draperies. Should either of these precautions be disregarded, insufficient heat is conducted away and the lamp bulb destroyed through internal overheating.

The first radiation should last three-quarters or a full hour, but with sensitive skins, as with children or fair-skinned women, caution is advisable at the commencement ; the first treatment should last only half-an-hour and the skin should be greased beforehand. When irradiating the face, the eyes must be protected. In all cases where irradiation is given after an operation without the use of a colour filter, no after-pain should follow.

Irradiation with the Sollux lamp is indicated in periodontitis and periostitis. It gives complete relief of pain, or at least great alleviation.

Hubert Müller, of Munich, used irradiation in cases of periodontitis, periostitis, pain following administration of arsenic, gingivitis, stomatitis, post-operative pain, and difficult dentition ; and was able to record good results after one to ten treatments.

In surgical procedure, luminous heat radiation acts as a valuable adjuvant in the following way :—Before the operation, and prior to injection, the area to be operated on is irradiated for half-an-hour with the blue filter. The effect of the resultant vasomotor contraction is to produce a condition of local anæmia, which both renders the field of treatment more accessible to view and strengthens the action of the novocain-suprarenalin solution. It is thus possible to produce deeper and longer local anæsthesia even with weaker injections. After the operation, a Sollux irradiation with clear light (no filter being used) should be given immediately. The antagonistic action of these rays results in early suspension of the existing anæsthesia, and the hyperæmia which is soon produced gives good local concentration of blood, so assisting prompt healing.

In treating ulcerous or pyogenic conditions in the area of the alveolar prolongations, the Sollux lamp is again an excellent adjuvant.

Dr. Phillip, of Dülken, obtained good results by this means in severe trismus.

R. Müller,* of Münster, obtained rapid dispersal of severe œdematous swellings by Sollux irradiations. In acute inflammatory conditions of the oral membrane, rapid resorptive action

*Deutsche zahnärztl. Wochenschr., No. 24, 1924.

took place in those cases where direct irradiation was possible. Müller also observed rapid absorption of drugs in the combined use of iodine, ' preso '-iodine, or phenol-camphor with luminous heat rays.

———————————

Ultra-violet therapy (with the quartz lamp) is therefore used in inflammatory and suppurative conditions in the mouth, and for treating scars in the oral cavity ; and hyperæmia therapy (with the Sollux lamp) in periodontitis, periostitis, pain after adminis-tration of arsenic, gingivitis, stomatitis, post-operative pain, difficult dentition, pyorrhœa alveolaris, facial and trigeminal neuralgia, and œdematous swellings.

Appendix.

RECENT CONTRIBUTIONS TO ULTRA-VIOLET THERAPY.

By Dr. Hugo Bach.

(*Strahlentherapie, Vol.* 34, 1929.)

In the use of artificial sources for light therapy, the works of Peemöller and Dannmeyer* may be accepted as having established clearly that only the Hanovia Alpine Sun quartz lamp can be seriously considered as an effective source of ultra-violet radiation. All other lamps (examined by them)† are much too weak in ultra-violet rays to produce the degree of erythema on the skin which is generally recognized as the measure of ultra-violet action. Non-evacuated quartz burners (so-called) have such great technical defects as compared with the evacuated Hanovia burners that they will soon disappear, as earlier experiments with such burners have already shown.

In the past, attempts were made to produce an artificial source of light giving the closest possible imitation of natural mountain sunlight in all its properties, its spectrum and its action ; to have red light and ultra-violet rays in the same proportion as in sunlight. Such a lamp would not, however, give any such intense ultra-violet rays as the Alpine Sun quartz lamp. It would necessitate very long exposures, which are impossible in practice. The obvious way is to use a source of heat rays, such as the Sollux Lamp, if the practitioner wishes to use both kinds of light simultaneously and with a reasonably short treatment period.

The action of ultra-violet rays on the organism as a whole consists in intensification of the natural vital processes (Ziegler).‡ In principle, he states, they increase function in the widest sense. Hörnicke§ describes this effect as actually a protein shock therapy similar to any other specific or non-specific protein therapy already

*M.Kl., 1923, No. 29. *Strahlentherapie*, vol. xxii., 1926.
†Inserted—(Translator).
‡*Strahlentherapie*, vol. xiv., 1922.
§*Strahlentherapie*, vol. xxviii., 1928.

referred to by Ostermann and others.* By varying dosage to individual requirements, Hörnicke, by using this protein-shock therapy, carried out courses for reducing or increasing the fat on obese or emaciated subjects respectively, as Wagner of Graz had previously done. In this regard it must be remembered that powerful and too frequent irradiations result in exciting nervous subjects, while mild and not too frequent treatments have a tranquillizing and refreshing effect.

This ultra-violet protein-shock therapy has been successfully used in many conditions; chronic arthritic, myopathic, and neuralgic cases; surgical tuberculosis, gouty deposits, alopecia, varicose ulcers, ulcerous gummata, etc. Recently Weiss† has recommended it for cases of sciatica which show no improvement under ordinary therapeutic methods. For successful results it is essential to obtain a dermatitis; this is harmless and soon passes off. The areas treated must always be small—the size of the palm—and intense erythema doses must be given.

There is another direction in which the chief action of ultra-violet rays is to intensify natural vital processes. This is the inwardly directed protective skin-function which Hoffmann‡ termed esophylaxis, and to which Bruno Bloch§ has also drawn attention.

Through this highly important biological function, these writers state, the vital internal organs are protected from disease bacteria, or have to deal, at most, with a relatively small and weakened part of these organisms. Bloch regards this capacity of the skin as one of the most important connections between dermatology and general medicine. His starting point lies in the results of recent investigations on allergy of the skin in trichophytosis, tuberculosis and syphilis. He emphasizes that the skin, above all other organs, plays an active part in the phenomena of allergy, immunity, and hyper-sensitivity; this is in strong contrast with the serum immunity produced in tetanus, diphtheria, etc., in which the blood acts as the carrier of the defensive forces. Hoffmann holds that the beneficial action of ultra-violet radiations on this

---

*Zeits. f. Erkrank des Bewegungsapparates, No. 2, 1924.

†M. Kl., 1929.

‡D.m.W., 1919, No. 45.

§Address at Zurich. (See also Prof. Memmesheimer's address, St. John's Hospital Dermatological Society, 18th Annual Report.—Translator.)

function is best explained by the assumption that they stimulate
a form of " internal secretion " of the epidermal epithelial cells,
and thus assist healing by promoting the increase of protective
substances.   Hesse* also holds it a proven and undeniable fact
that in the most varied acute and chronic processes, particularly
syphilis, healing is accelerated by light, *i.e.* by irradiation of the
skin-organ for which light is the appropriate stimulus.   " We
must," says he, " turn our attention more to immunization by
light." No experimental data are available on immunization by
light, but practical experience teaches that human resistance to
infection is specially increased by ultra-violet radiation.   Among
others, Donnelly has called attention to this from observation on
a large number of cases.   It should therefore be a fruitful field for
exact investigation, to put the question of immunization against
infectious diseases by ultra-violet light on to a scientific basis.

As with all other physical treatments applied to the skin, the
field of use for ultra-violet rays is very wide, since any causes
affecting the physiological functions of the skin also affect the
various disturbances in bodily economy.   A great variety of internal
and external diseases are treated successfully by irradiation, so long
as no fever is present.

Ultra-violet light thus serves not only as a direct means of
healing, as in rickets and tetany, but also as an adjuvant and
roborant, *e.g.* in weakness, conditions of exhaustion and convalescence.   It is in addition successfully used by the healthy as
a prophylactic and tonic agency to maintain and improve health.
In this regard it may well be reckoned one of the ordinary hygienic
measures such as air and sun baths, exercise, sports and hydro-
therapeutic measures of every kind.

According to numerous reports by doctors and trainers, ultra-
violet irradiations increase the athletic powers.   Both in England
and Germany doctors have recommended the use of these rays in
schools, pointing out that children receiving regular ultra-violet
radiation are more active in mind and body, and more resistant
to disease than those not irradiated.

Among numerous indications for treatment, only a few of the
more recent are here mentioned.   Hufnagel† found that ultra-
violet rays frequently have a directly abortive action in influenza.

Strahlentherapie, vol. xii., 1926.

†*Mm. W.*, 1928, No. 32.

Hörnicke* observed increased resistance to disease after irradiation, and recommends it as a prophylactic measure against influenza. Voute and Jost† state that irradiation is the best although not the only cure for frostbite. Kühne recommends ultra-violet irradiation almost to an erythema degree against freckles, and as a prophylactic against sunburn and glacier burn. I. Spiro‡ reports good results from ultra-violet radiations in eye diseases of the young ; blepharitis, conjunctivitis, phlyctenular kerato-conjunctivitis, phlyctenular keratitis, corneal ulceration and tuberculous iritis. These eye diseases seen in young people are mostly due to rickets, tuberculosis or under-nourishment, in all probability not a deficiency of food but of sunlight. He states that ultra-violet irradiation is the most effective and best-known remedy for these " deficiency diseases." These eye conditions usually heal up under general treatment alone, without local treatment ; the latter must, however, not be neglected, but should be left to the specialist.

Dosage for ultra-violet rays is variously stated by different authors. This is not surprising in view of the variations in the human skin resulting in different individual reactions to ultra-violet light. Furthermore individual dosage is necessary with irradiation as with every other therapy ; it is most important to find the correct erythema dosage in individual cases. The works of Behring, and of Rost-Keller, give further information on this point, and Keller's erythema dosimeter will be found useful. Full data and dosage are given in the present work.

Ultra-violet light acts on animals and plants as on man. It promotes their growth and they thrive better in all respects with irradiation than without. All these observations seem to indicate that all life on the earth is due chiefly to the action of the short-waved rays.

At the other end of the spectrum from the short-waved, cold ultra-violet rays, we find the long-waved red and infra-red rays which carry heat. In his work on quartz light, Thedering points out that these two ends of the spectrum, the red and the violet are also " antagonistic " in their energy characteristics ; the red is warm, chemically inactive, mentally exciting ; the violet cold, chemically and biologically active, mentally soothing. This

*Strahlentherapie, vol. xxviii., 1928.
†Schweizer Med. Wschr., No. 52, 1920.
‡British Journal of Actinotherapy, June, 1928.

" antagonism " would argue that ultra-violet inflammation, including sunburn, can be subdued by red light, which is actually the case. Red light treatment should therefore be carried out in a dark room, since the violet must be excluded. Ludwig and von Ries* were able to show that the luminescence of phosphorescent screens was excited by ultra-violet, violet or blue, but extinguished by red and infra-red rays. Experiments on animals and plants showed that it is possible, by means of red light, to reverse Vitamin D activation effected by ultra-violet. Subsequent ultra-violet irradiation will again activate vitamin D after its extinction by red light.

Various authorities have lately written on ocular injuries caused by ultra-violet rays. Many years ago Schanz and Chalupecky surmised that protracted action of these rays caused lenticular opacity, and resulted in glass-blower's cataract ; English authorities, however, showed that glass-blower's cataract was not caused by ultra-violet but by infra-red rays. It has long been known, as Birch-Hirschfeld† writes, that ultra-violet rays have a strong inflammatory action on the anterior parts of the eye, the conjunctiva and the cornea ; i.e., their effects are developed in those parts where they are strongly absorbed, causing " photophthalmia electrica." He considers it indubitable that the middle spectrum region, i.e., the visible rays, may, at great intensity, also be injurious to the vital parts of the eye, and adds the remark that many now believed the infra-red to be the only harmful rays, and considered the ultra-violet quite innocuous to the interior of the eye.

Bückler.‡ of the Berlin University Eye Clinic, has published the following results of his investigations on the effects of highly concentrated infra-red and ultra-violet rays on the eye :—

The shorter infra-red (1500-800 A.U.) produces after only half-an-hour's exposure, fibrinous exudation into the aqueous humour, iridocyclitis with hyaline degeneration of the iris stroma, and rarefication of the posterior pigment layer. In the lens, vacuolation occurs, with extensive destruction of fibres in the anterior and posterior parts of the sclerotic. The retina and choroid are also severely affected. With isolated ultra-violet rays down to about

---

*Strahlentherapie, vol. xxix., 1928.

†Med. Welt., 1929, No. 23.

‡Kl. W., 1929, No. 17.

2850 A.U., even after exposures of several hours, the only changes noted were transitory vacuolation in the corneal epithelium, and passing exudation into the aqueous humour; but no trace of opacity in the lens or damage to the retina. This is in accordance with the known fact that ultra-violet rays penetrate 0·5 mm. at most, and cannot therefore penetrate into the interior of the eye. Practical experience also teaches that, apart from photophthalmia electrica, ultra-violet rays have never been observed to cause any injury to the eye, particularly the internal parts. Although the photophthalmia electrica usually heals spontaneously within a few days without treatment, it is advisable to protect the eyes from ultra-violet radiation by means of goggles.

Trendtel* recommends as a protection against ultra-violet rays (particularly wave-lengths 2800-2600) drops of corodenin (0·3% solution of 5 ethoxychinolin, 8 sulphacid of formula $C_2 H_5 OSO_3 HN$, produced by Reidel dé Haen of Berlin).

On the therapeutic action of light this necessarily brief summary of recent research shows that the various rays of sunlight, the source of all life on earth, can be utilized in medicine in most diverse directions; but that the ultra-violet rays are outstanding in their far-reaching effects, both in health and disease. We cannot fathom their nature, yet further exact research will throw more and more light on their effect on mankind, animals and plants.

*Med. Welt., 1929, No. 22.

INDEX OF AUTHORITIES

INDEX OF SUBJECTS

215